AF480039

Pharmaceutical Dosage Form

Basics and Beyond...

Second Edition

Pharmaceutical Dosage Form

Basics and Beyond...

Second Edition

Kamlesh J. Wadher
Professor
Smt. Kishoritai Bhoyar College of Pharmacy, Kamptee

Milind J. Umekar
Professor and Principal
Smt. Kishoritai Bhoyar College of Pharmacy, Kamptee

and

Mahesh R. Mishra
Associate Professor
Smt. Kishoritai Bhoyar College of Pharmacy, Kamptee

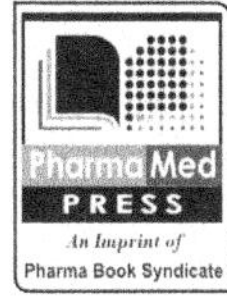

PharmaMed Press
An imprint of Pharma Book Syndicate
A unit of BSP Books Pvt. Ltd.
4-4-309/316, Giriraj Lane,
Sultan Bazar, Hyderabad - 500 095.

Pharmaceutical Dosage Form : *Basics and Beyond..., Second Edition*
by Kamlesh J. Wadher, Milind J. Umekar and Mahesh R. Mishra

© 2019, 2017, *by Publisher*
Second Edition 2019

Published by

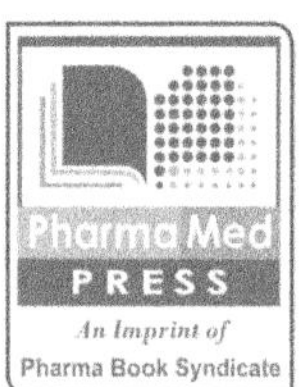

PharmaMed Press

An imprint of Pharma Book Syndicate

A unit of BSP Books Pvt. Ltd.

4-4-309/316, Giriraj Lane, Sultan Bazar, Hyderabad - 500 095.
Phone: 040-23445688, 23445600; Fax: 91+40-23445611
E-mail: info@pharmamedpress.com
www.pharmamedpress.com/pharmamedpress.net

ISBN: 978-93-88305-22-8 (Hardback)

Preface

The textbook ***Pharmaceutical* Dosage Form : *Basics and Beyond...,* *Second Edition*** is written with the basic objective to cover various important aspects of pharmaceutical dosage form including, pre-formulation, formulation, recent technological advancements and packaging in an integrated approach. Although several books are available on the individual dosage form; we tried to present simple, concise and appropriate book for the students as well as teachers of pharmaceutical science.

As this book is written for pharmacy graduates and post graduate students we have also included basic concepts in the developments of various pharmaceutical dosage forms to make it more useful resource for the budding pharmacist. We have covered all the established dosage forms in 12 different chapters with separate sub sections and simplified with schematic presentation wherever necessary.

The concept of preformulation including the need of dosage form is depicted in chapter 1. The formulation of solid dosage form such as tablets, tablet coating, capsules and microencapsulation techniques are represented in chapter 2, 3 and 4 respectively. These chapters particularly deals with excipients and methods used to prepare them, and its evaluation. Chapter 5 described pharmaceutical importance and techniques of microencapsulation. The formulations of liquids orals as, solution, suspensions and emulsions including their required theoretical aspects are presented in Chapter 6. In chapter 7 presented, formulation of semisolid dosage forms (creams, ointments). Chapter 8 described the manufacturing aspects of parenteral formulations including the considerations of tonicity and sterility. The formulation of Aerosol as metered-dose system is presented in chapter 9. The formulation of ophthalmic dosage form is described in Chapter 10. In addition to the description of ocular formulations, this chapter concisely describes the absorption constraints for ocular delivery of drugs. Chapter 11 described the formulation of suppositories particularly emphasizing on the various factors affecting rectal absorption of drugs. Packaging aspects of dosage form including types, specifications and methods of evaluation are depicted in chapter 12. Beyond this we have included recent advancements in pharmaceutical dosage form. Chapter 13 described Cosmetics.

The primary objective of this book is to provide updated knowledge and skills required for the formulation of dosage form. The key assets of the book are simple and easy to understand language, incorporation of tables and figures to make each chapter more precise and interesting. We hope that students as well as teachers will gain a comprehensive understanding of formulation aspects to formulate different dosage forms.

We are grateful to the managements of Shri Sadashivrao Patil Sikshan Sanstha, Kamptee for all the support and encouragement for this writing. We are obliged and gratified to our family without their patience and support the book would not have been completed.

Key Features

- Provides an integrated approach explaining pre-formulation and formulation aspects of various dosage form.

- Emphasize on the basic pharmaceutical concepts, its principles and technologies applied in the manufacturing of pharmaceutical dosages and drug delivery systems.

- Beyond the basics, it covers recent advancement and trends in dosage forms technology.

-Authors

Contents

Chapter 3   Tablet Coating

Chapter 7   Semisolid Dosage Forms

Chapter 8   Parenteral Products

Chapter 9   Pharmaceutical Aerosols

Chapter 11 Suppositories

1 Dosage Form Design

An important milestone in the drug development process is the discovery of an active compound, which is a long and multifaceted process. The evolution of new chemical entity has vastly increased over the last few decades mainly because of the commencement of high throughput methods for drug synthesis and screening. Drug development primarily involves investigations on 'lead molecules' identified in drug discovery stage. A lead compound has to voyage through a series of investigations and experimentations to provide a researcher early efficacy and safety evaluation.

Ideally drugs must be, properly absorbed into the systemic circulation, distributed to the proper site of action, metabolized efficiently and effectively, excreted well from the body and should be not toxic. Preformulation studies help researchers scrutinize lead compounds early in the discovery process. The lead molecule is used to generate specific chemical compounds with the optimal physiochemical, pharmaceutical, pharmacokinetics, pharmacodynamic, pharmacological and safety characteristics. The potential for these features can be predicted from reasonably interim preclinical and clinical studies and for the proper and speedy drug development, it is obligatory to select a compound with favourable pharmaceutical and pharmacological properties.

A new compound after its identification has to undergo a complete procedure of drug development before it can be transformed into its proper dosage form. It is important to characterize physicochemical, pharmacodynamic properties and pharmacological screening of the new drug substance for the development of safe and sound dosage forms. The objectives of formulation development are to ensure accurate dose and dosing regimen to present the drug substance in a convenient form for the patient and to increase the stability of the drug to prolong its shelf-life.

Drugs are hardly ever administered alone; they are always and preferably given in the form of formulated preparations due to different physical, chemical and biological constraints. To provide some basic pharmaceutical functions, drugs or chemical substances are administered as a component of formulation in combination with one or more additives. Transforming a drug into a proper dosage form not only provides various advantages like ease of handling, ease of administration, better stability but may also lead to better therapeutic efficacy and bioavailability.

A dosage form is defined as a physical form of a drug such as a solid, liquid, or gas by which it is delivered in its proper form to particular sites of action within the body. Common dosage forms include solutions, tablets, capsules, semisolids, injections, and aerosols. The proper designing and formulation of any dosage form requires consideration of the physical, chemical, and biologic characteristics of the drug moiety and additives to be used in formulating the product.

Dosage form is necessary because there are certain conditions where only particular route of administration is feasible or preferable. In case of dysphasia, nausea and vomiting, oral administration is not suitable and one has to opt for other routes such as parenteral, topical or inhalation. Similarly, in case of joint pain, local application or topical route is preferable.

Pharmaceutics can be defined as an area of study concerned with the formulation, fabrication, stability, and efficacy of pharmaceutical dosage forms. There must be compatibility between drug and pharmaceutical additives to make a stable, efficacious, attractive, easy to administer, safe and sound pharmaceutical product. The product should be manufactured in strict quality control which contributes to its stability. The product should be properly packaged and stored under appropriate conditions that contribute to maximum shelf life.

1.1   Characteristics of Ideal Dosage Form

Dosage forms are pharmaceutical products that involve combination of active drug and non-drug substances, along with other non recoverable materials. Drug needs to be in the most convenient and proper form, so that it reaches to the desired site of action, which is greatly influenced by the types of dosage form of the drug. There are various types of dosage forms available which are used in accord with a particular reason; as on the basis of characteristics and advantage.

Many factors specify the characteristics of an ideal dosage form. Ideal Dosage Form should be:

- Easy and safe to administer
- Easy to handle

- Easy to reproduce and manufacture
- High patient compliance
- Efficacious
- Physically and chemically stable
- Biocompatible
- Economical to the patient
- Maintain its therapeutic activity throughout the shelf life

1.2   The Need for Dosage Forms

Drug substances hardly are ever taken without adding additives, due to difficulty in taking precise amount of dose and the desired therapeutic effect may not be obtained. The drug and excipients are suitably compounded to convert them into various suitable dosage forms such as solution, tablets, capsules, suspensions, emulsions, ointments, paste etc. The selection and processing of excipients are as equally important as the selection of drugs alone as it may alter the therapeutic properties of drug (Figure 1.1). By controlling the organoleptic properties using suitable additives such as colours, flavors etc. patient acceptability can be enhanced Dosage form provides desired therapeutic level of a drug.

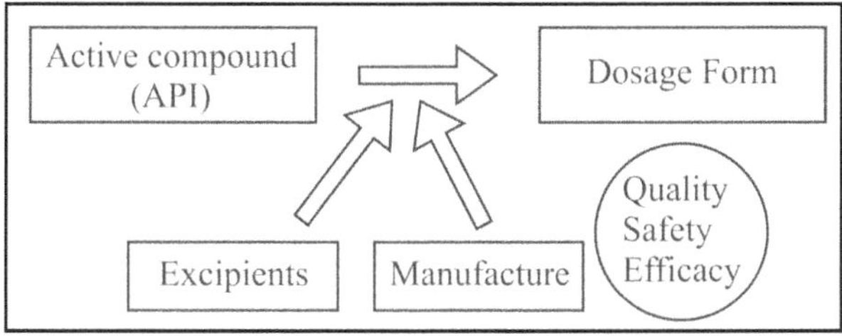

FIGURE 1.1 Flow chart of need for dosage form.

For a potent and low dose drug it could be difficult for the patients to take appropriate and exact dose of a drug from the bulk material. Most drug substances available for use are administered in milligram and micrograms, which are too small to weigh.

It is impossible for a patient to obtain exact amount from a bulk supply (100 mg) of Diclofenac sodium. How could one weigh Levothyroxine with dose 0.1 mg. When the dose of a drug is small, it will lead to patient inconvenience.

TABLE 1.1

Dose of some drugs

Drug	Usual dose (mg)	Category
Ethynyl estradiol	0.05	Estrogen
Levothyroxin	0.10	Antiulcerative
Digoxin	0.25	Cardiotonic
Nitroglycerine	0.40	Antianginal
Alprazolam	0.50	Antianxiety
Clonazepam	1.00	Anticonvulsant
Aripiprazole	2	Antipsycotic
Estropiate	1.25	Estrogen
Risperidone	2.00	Antipsycotic
Prazosine HCL	2.00	Antihypertensive
Lisinopril	5	Antihypertensive
Chlorpheniramine maleate	4	Antihistaminic
Naltraxone	4.5	Multiple sclerosis
Enalapril Maleate	5	Antihypertensive
Omeprazol	10	Antiulcerative
Nifedapine	10	Vasodilator

When the dose of the drug is less as is with so many drugs (Table 1.1), a suitable dosage form such as tablets or capsules should be prepared by adding bulking agents (diluents) to make dosage form sufficient enough to handle properly. The overall objective of dosage form design is to increase the stability of the drug substance to extend its shelf life, ensure accurate dosing and to deliver the drug in a suitable form.

1.3   Primary Reasons for Designing a Dosage Form

A. Protection

1. To protect the drug from the external environmental conditions such as, atmospheric oxygen, temperature and humidity (coated tablets, capsules, ampoules)
2. To prevent degradation of acid labile drug from gastric acid in the stomach (Enteric-coated)

B. Improve Therapeutic Activity

1. To provide optimal drug action to the appropriate site (ointments, creams, transdermal patches)
2. Placement of drugs directly in the body's orifices (rectal, vaginal suppositories)
3. To provide optimal drug action in the bloodstream or body tissues (injections, inhalants, inhalation aerosols)
4. To provide rate controlled drug action (prolonged release delivery)
5. To improve bioavailability of drug with narrow absorption window (gastroretentive delivery)

C. Patient Compliance

1. Accuracy of dose by providing unit dose (tablets, capsules)
2. Reduction in frequency of dosing (sustained and prolonged release delivery)
3. Masking the bitter and unpleasant taste or odour of the drug. (Film coated tablets, Capsules, suspension, emulsion)
4. Placement of drugs within body tissues and cavities (otic, rectal, vaginal, buccal, sublingual)
5. Ease of handling and administration (chewable tablets)

1.4 Types of Dosage Form

Depending on the physical form, and route of administration, dosage forms can be classified as shown in Table 1.2.

A. On the basis of Physical Form

1. Solid dosage form

E.g. conventional and modified release tablets, powders, capsules, films, lozenges, chewing gum, pellets.

2. Liquid dosage form

E.g. solution, syrup, elixir, spirit, aromatic water, tincture, injections, mouth washes gargles, suspension, emulsion.

3. Semisolid dosage form

Semisolid dosage form used for the application to the skin and mucous membrane (otic, nasal, vaginal, or rectal). *E.g.* ointment, cream, gel, liniment, lotions, and pastes.

4. Gaseous dosage form

Combination of an active ingredient with propellant which upon actuation emits a fine dispersion of liquid and/or solid materials in a gaseous medium *E.g.* aerosol, inhaler, nebulizer.

B. On the basis of Route of Administration

1. Oral-through oral route

- Powder
- Tablet-buccal, sub lingual, or orally disintegrating, modified release.
- Capsule-Hard gelatin and soft gels
- Liquids–Monophasic and Biphasic

2. Topical-applied over the skin surface and mucosa

- Cream, gel, liniment or balm, lotion, or ointment, etc.
- Ear drops (otic)
- Eye drops (ophthalmic)
- Skin patch (transdermal)
- Vaginal rings

3. Parenteral-applied through the skin

- Intradermal (ID) Injection in the dermal region
- Intramuscular (IM) injection directly into a muscle
- Intraosseous (IO) injection directly into the marrow of a bone
- Intravenous (IV) is the infusion or injection of liquid drug directly into a vein
- Subcutaneous (SC) is the administration as a bolus into the subcutaneous layer
- Intrathecal (IT) Injection into the spinal column

4. Inhalational

- Instilled through the nasal and pulmonary route
  E.g. aerosol, inhale, nebulizer

5. Instilled in the body cavities

Suppository, douche, pessary etc.,

- Rectal
- Vaginal

TABLE 1.2

Dosage forms with their merits and demerits

Types of dosage form	Merits	Demerits
Solid dosage forms: Tablets, Capsules, Lozenges, Chewing gum, Pellets, Films	1. Dose accuracy 2. Stability of the drug 2. Portability 3. Uniformity of dose 4. Reproducibility 5. High Mechanical strength 6. Tamper resistance 6. Masking of taste, odour 7. Easy to pack, handling and transportation	1. Not suitable for unconscious patient 2. Patient non compliance due to difficulty in swallowing (Dysphasia) 2. Formulation complications 3. Not preferable for acid labile and stomach irritant drugs.
Liquid dosage forms **Monophasic:** Solutions, Elixir, Syrups, **Biphasic:** Suspensions, Emulsions	1. Easy to swallow 2. Easy to manufacture 3. Fast absorption 4. Improves bioavailability 5. Less processing steps 6. Less excipients required as compared to tablets	1. Non uniformity of dose. 2. Prone to microbial attack 3. Bulky 4. More chances of loss by the breakage during shipping and transportation 5. Unsuitable for unpleasant taste and obnoxious odour drugs 6. Less stability
Semisolid dosage forms: Cream, Gel, Liniment , Lotion, or Ointment, etc	1. Easy to use. 2. More stable than liquid dosage form. 3. Avoidance of first pass metabolism 4. Local action of drug on affected area 5. Patient convenience (easy to apply and remove)	1. Difficult to handle. 2. Chances of contamination (Application with finger) 3. More prone to environment effect. 4. May cause staining and irritation.
Gaseous dosage form	1. Easy to handle and convenient 2. Withdrawal of dose without Contamination 3. Environmental protection of unstable drug 4. Provides medication to local area 5. Dose adjustment possible (metered valves) 6. Tamper proof	1. Expensive 2. May create environmental Hazards 3. Dosing not reproducible 4. Non Reliable performance 5. Limited safety.

1.5 General Considerations in Dosage Form Design

- Preformulation studies
- Drug and Drug Product Stability

For rational design of the dosage forms, preformulation is an important development step used to characterize the properties of drug substance and also to understand the challenges that a particular compound may possess during the formulation. It helps to optimize both the preclinical and clinical development with fast and high quality delivery of drug product in the proper dosage forms.

1.5.1 Preformulation Concept

After drug discovery, with a knowledge based on physical, chemical and biopharmaceutical properties of the drug molecule, the foremost aim of pharmaceutical scientist is to formulate drug in the suitable form which improves patient compliance and that is apt for easy administration. All the activities carried out at and before formulation stage of dosage form, are collectively called as pre-formulation studies. It helps to understand the concept of formulation development on a scientific basis. It is a requisite to characterize physical and chemical properties of drug before the formulation and development into a dosage form.

Preformulation testing includes all studies performed on a newly identified drug substance in order to produce a stable and therapeutically effective drug dosage form. Thus, initial learning phase related to drug is known as pre-formulation. This information provides an outline for the drugs combination with additives in the manufacturing of a robust dosage form.

The consideration of the physical, chemical, and biological characteristics of drug substance and excipients to be used in formulating the dosage form is utmost necessary for the appropriate design and formulation of the dosage form. Preformulation also involves the application of pharmacokinetic and biopharmaceutical principles to the physicochemical properties of drug substance with the aim of designing most favourable drug delivery (safe, effective, and stable) system. Preformulation is the border line between development of new drug substances and formulation development. It helps to endow road map for full formulation and development.

Before beginning the proper pre-formulation studies, it is important to glance into the following factors:

- Innovative molecule or abbreviated
- Therapeutic category of drug compound
- Amount of drug substance available
- Physicochemical properties of the drug
- Physicochemical properties of excipient and possible interaction with drug
- Therapeutic dose/potency of a compound
- The category of dosage form to be prepared
- Stability parameters

1.5.2 Goal of Preformulation

A comprehensive understanding of the properties of the newly synthesized drug substance helps to minimize problems related to the later stages of formulation and development; reduces the overall cost of formulation and development, and curtail the time required for complete development of drug product.

The goals of preformulation studies are:

1. Selection of correct form of the drug substance (solid, liquid, gas) based on a type of dosage form development
2. Evaluation of physical and chemical properties of drug substance
3. To understand biopharmaceutical properties of drug
4. To reduce drug development time and cost
5. To produce safe, effective and reproducible drug delivery system

Three factors drive the preformulation studies:

1. Regulatory requirements,
2. Commercial requirements and
3. Technological development

1.5.3 Significance of Preformulation Study

It is a process of designing the drug delivery thorough determination of physical, and chemical properties of newly synthesized drug molecule and it provide useful information for subsequent formulation of a physicochemically stable and biopharmaceutically suitable dosage form. Preformulation study helps to:

- Establish the new drug molecule's identity
- Characterize physicochemical properties of new drug molecule.
- Determine drug and excipients compatibility
- Correlate pharmacokinetics and biopharmaceutical properties.
- Establish kinetic rate profile of new drug
- Optimize preclinical and clinical process
- Provide necessary data for development of analytical methods
- Produce safe, innovative, stable cost effective dosage form.

Data from preformulation studies minimizes problems in various phases of drug development and provides critical foundation for the successful formulation effort and thus reducing the overall cost of development of product

Preformulation factors include physical properties such as particle size, crystalline structure, melting point, solubility, partition coefficient, dissolution, membrane permeability, dissociation constants, and drug stability. For successful development of any formulation various factors need to be considered such as the type of drug and excipients, compatibility, storage condition selection of containers, packaging, stability and patient compliance such as, considerations of organoleptic properties i.e., taste, appearance, odour and palatability.

These preformulation investigations provide a rationale for the design of proper formulation and support the need for the drugs modification (salts formation, prodrug, and chemical modification) for the effective and reproducible product development with maximum bioavailability. Alterations in drug substance are carried out for improvements of certain pharmaceutical properties as shown in Table 1.3.

TABLE 1.3

Improvement of pharmaceutical properties

Pharmaceutical properties	Examples
Solubility enhancement	Doxycycline, Erythromycin
Stability	Cephalexin, Theophylline
Prolonged action	Heptominol, Alkylbiguanide
Reduce toxicity	Bephenium, Kanamycin
Improve organoleptic properties	Vincamine, Propoxyphene
Activity enhancement	Tetracycline, Propoxyphene
Absorption	Aspirin, Ampicillin

Salt form modification is restricted to ionisable molecules. Alternately, for molecular drug prodrugs may be formed. Prodrugs are synthetic derivatives of drug molecules which liberate parent molecules *in vivo* after some modification. Erythromycin is a bitter taste drug and is hydrolyzed in gastric acid. This problem can be solved by preparing a prodrug of parent molecules, Erythromycin estolate.

1.5.4 Preformulation Types

Preformulation can be broadly classified into two classes as depicted in Table 1.4.

Fundamental Properties: Properties which are dependent on the chemical structure and surface morphology of the drug molecule which include:

(a) **Solubility:** Solubility parameters in different solvents, pH solubility profile, dissociation constant (pK_a) of drug, salt formation, partition or distribution coefficient (log P or log D), and dissolution kinetics

(b) **Permeability**

(c) **Solid state properties:** solid form, polymorphism, solvated forms and amorphous form

(d) **Stability:** Solid state and solution state stability, inherent stability, pH stability profile and photo stability

Derived Properties: These properties are derived from the fundamental properties which include:

(a) Characterization of particle properties like morphology, particle size and shape

(b) Bulk density, tap density

(c) Flow properties

(d) Compaction behaviour: Hausner ratio and Carr's Index

(e) Drug-excipient compatibility

TABLE 1.4

Preformulation drug characterization properties

Fundamental properties	Derived properties
Samples assay by UV spectroscopy	Particle size and size distribution-Microscopy
Solubility - Aqueous, pKa, Salt, Solvents, Partition coefficient, Dissolution	Bulk density
Melting point	Flow properties
Assay development	Compression properties
Stability in solution and solid state	Drug- excipient compatibility

Bulk characterization

(a)   Physical description: Particle size and surface characterization

(b)   Crystal properties and polymorphism

(c)   Hygroscopycity

(d)   Purity: Melting point depression

(e)   Flowability

Solubility analysis

(a)   Solubility

(b)   Ionization constant (pK_a)

(c)   Partition coefficient

(d)   Dissolution

(e)   Common ion effect

Stability analysis

(a)   Solid state

(b)   Solution state

(c)   Compatibility

1.5.4.1 Bulk Characterization

During the process development, bulk properties of the drug substance such as particle size, crystallinity, powder flow, compaction case, melting point and other physical characteristics influence the final dosage form during the preformulation stage.

(a) *Physical Description*: **Particle Size and Surface Characterization:** Bulk properties of the formulation differ from pure drug. But these properties do not change for solid form of drug. Each new drug candidate has to be tested for particle size and shape during preformulation study as with the smaller particle size it is impractical to make possible uniform and homogenous formulation. Various physicochemical and bio-pharmaceutical properties of drug substances are affected by their particle size distribution and shapes.

The particle size and size distribution characteristics of the drug have a large impact on its rate of delivery in the body. As a part of the drug validation process the regulatory agencies have a stringent requirement for determining the chemical and physical characteristics of drug particles.

Surface characteristics of a drug play a fundamental role in determining both bulk powder and suspension properties. The most important physical property of particulate samples is particle size and shape as they have a direct influence on material properties such as, dissolution rate. (Tablets), stability (Suspension), efficacy of delivery (Aerosols), appearance, packing, density and porosity (powder), texture feel (topical), flowability, handling (granules), and viscosity (semisolids).

The particle size and distribution of drug substance and excipients have significant and potential effects on the quality of the final dosage form, like product colour, appearance, mixing, flowability, solubility, dissolution, bioavailability, stability, content uniformity, compressibility, drying, packaging and quality control. Particle size and distribution analysis of a sample can be performed using a variety of techniques, both qualitative and quantitative.

There are many different methods available for particle size analysis such as:

- Sieving
- Sedimentation
- Optical microscopy
- Electron microscopy
- Coulter counter
- Laser diffractometers.

Microscopy and sedimentation are the simplest technique of determining size distribution and shapes, but shortcoming include being slow and tedious for quantitative determination. Sieving is less practical technique due to lack of bulk material at preformulation stage. Coulter counter and Laser diffractometers techniques are becoming more popular due to advantages such as, rapid counting, flexibility, reliability and used for the wide range of sizes.

Surface morphology may be determined by scanning electron microscopy (SEM) technique, atomic force microscopy (AFM) and Scanning tunneling microscopy (STM) which precisely gives qualitatively determination of shape and surface area of particles. SEM uses a focused beam of high-energy electrons to generate a variety of signals at the surface of solid specimen. It is technique where only few milligram quantity of material is used to determine particle size, shape and texture, but having disadvantage that it unable to characterizing finer particles and agglomerates. AFM has several advantages over the SEM. Unlike the electron microscope which provides a two-dimensional image of a sample, the AFM provides a three-dimensional surface profile. In a very short time this technique is helpful to collect significant data on the size and morphology of the particles.

Laser diffraction spectroscopy, is a technique that utilizes diffraction patterns of a laser beam passed through any object to measure geometrical dimensions of the particle. The techniques are based on the diffraction theory, which states that the intensity of light scattered by a particle is directly proportional to the particle size. The various techniques used to estimate particle size with their ability of determining the size range is depicted in the Table 1.5.

TABLE 1.5

Particle size techniques and size range

Method	Size range (μ)
Sieving (woven wire)	20–125,000
optical Microscopy	0.5–150
electron Microscopy	0.001–5
Sedimentation	0.1–50
Coulter counter	1–200
Laser diffractometers	0.001–1

- ***Surface Area Determination***

   Surface area is most commonly determined by gas adsorption method based on Brunaver, Emette and Teller (BET) theory of nitrogen adsorption. Most substances adsorb a mono molecular layer of gas under certain conditions of partial pressure of gas and temperature. Knowing the monolayer capacity of adsorbent and the area of absorbable molecule, the surface area can be calculated.

(b) ***Crystal Properties and Polymorphism***: Polymorphism is the property of a solid material to exist in two or more different molecular arrangements or crystalline structures of the same chemical compound. A polymorph is a solid material with two or more different molecular arrangements giving distinct crystal species. Solid drug materials generally occur as amorphous and crystalline. Stability and pharmacological activity of drug substance greatly depends on its amorphous or crystalline nature. Amorphous drugs have randomly arranged atoms or molecules. They have higher thermodynamic energy, solubility and dissolution rate than corresponding crystalline form. But, during the various stages of processing and storage, they tend to change to more stable form. Crystals are characterized by repetitious arrangements of the constituent atoms in a regular three dimensional structure. Crystalline forms of drugs may be more preferable than the corresponding amorphous form because of greater stability. For example, sodium salt of crystalline forms of Penicillin G is more stable and has better therapeutic activity than corresponding amorphous forms.

Crystal habit and the internal structure of a drug is found to affect various properties such as, flowability, solubility, dissolution and stability. Habit is the description of the outer appearance of a crystal whereas the internal structure is the molecular arrangement within the solid. A single internal structure for a compound may have several different habits, depending on the environment of crystal growth.

Many drug substances which exist in more than one crystalline from with different space lattice arrangements are known as polymorphs and generally have different morphology, solubility, dissolution, tensile strength, density and melting points.

Polymorphism may be of two types

Enantiotropic: One polymorph reversibly changes into another form by a change in temperature and pressure, *e.g.*, Sulphur.

Monotropic: One polymorphic form is unstable at all temperatures and pressures *e.g.*, glyceryl stearates.

A drug substance may exist in two or more polymorphic forms but, only one form is found to be thermodynamically stable at a given temperature and pressure. The other forms would convert to the stable form with the progress of time. The stable polymorph exhibits the highest melting point, the lowest solubility, and the maximum chemical stability. Chloramphenicol exists in three polymorphic forms A, B and C, in which B form is found to be most stable.

Parameters to be considered during polymorphism study are: number and type of polymorphs, solubility parameters, degree of stability, stability of metastable form, temperature stability range, effect of processing conditions like drying, milling, micronization etc.,

Crystalline Nature and Polymorphism can be Measured by

Various Methods used to study crystalline nature and polymorphism, such as, microscopy, Fourier Transform Infrared Spectrometer (FT-IR), Differential scanning calorimeter (DSC), X-ray powder diffraction (XRD), thermal analysis, and dilalometry. Investigation of polymorphism and crystal habit of a drug substance during preformulation is essential as it relates greatly to the pharmaceutical processing.

(c) *Hygroscopicity*: Like many other substances, water soluble salt form of drugs has a tendency to absorb atmospheric moisture. Such types of materials can be classified as:

Hygroscopic material is which has a tendency to absorb moisture and get in equilibrium with water in the atmosphere.

Deliquescent substance is which partially or wholly liquefies after absorbing moisture from atmosphere.

Efflorescent substance is which has a tendency to loose water and becomes anhydrous.

Importance of hygroscopicity in preformulation

High susceptibility for moisture absorption leads to various processing related problems such as poor flow, weight variation, cracking, picking, sticking, handling problem, particle agglomeration and stability related problems such as, chemical breakdown, cake formation and colour change on storage.

Hygroscopicity can be measured by

1. *Dynamic vapour sorption method*: It is a gravimetric technique that measures the amount of a solvent which is absorbed by powder.

2. *Isothermal microcalorimetry*: This method is used for the determination of the critical relative humidity.

(d) *Purity: Melting Point Depression*: The melting point of a solid is the temperature at which the material changes from a solid to a liquid state i.e. solid in equilibrium with liquid state under an external pressure of one atmosphere. This physical property plays a vital role in preformulation phase to identify and characterize a drug substance.

Melting point can be measured by

The melting point of a drug can be measured using three techniques such as, capillary melting, hot stage microcopy and differential scanning calorimetric or thermal analysis.

Capillary melting: Drug substance is placed in a thin walled capillary tube closed at one end and heated slowly and evenly. The temperature at which the sample is observed to melt is taken as the melting point. Capillary melting gives information about the melting range.

Hot Stage Microcopy: Also known as Thermal microscopy where melting process is observed with the help of a microscope equipped with a heated and wrapped sample stage. It enables to study and characterize material physically as a function of temperature and time.

Differential Scanning Calorimetric and Differential Thermal Analysis

Differential scanning calorimetry (DSC) is a thermo analytical technique in which the difference in the amount of heat required to increase the temperature of a sample and reference is measured as a function of temperature. Both the sample and reference are maintained at nearly the same temperature throughout the experiment.

Differential thermal analysis (DTA) measures the temperature difference between the sample and a reference as a function of temperature or time when heating at a constant rate. In this technique it is the heat flow to the sample and reference that remains the same rather than the temperature.

Powder Flow Properties: Powder flow determination is crucial for the pharmaceutical manufacturing process. Powders are classified as free flowing or cohesive. Flow properties of the powder affected by a small variation on particle size, shape, density electro static charge and moisture level which ultimately affect the processing parameters. A powder flow investigation helps to assess an improvement in various stages of the formulation developments.

There are various methods available to measure the powder flow, which, include measurement of angle of repose, bulk density, tapped density, Carr's compressibility index and Hausner ratio.

- ***Angle of Repose***

  It is most important tool for estimation of flow property of powder. Determination is done by "fixed height funnel method" The angle of repose is the maximum angle which is formed between the horizontal base of the surface and the pile of the powder.

  The angle of repose (θ) was calculated as follows:

$$\tan\theta = \frac{h}{r}$$

  where, h = height of the pile

  r = radius of base of pile

- ***Carr's Compressibility Index and Hausner Ratio***

  Carr's compressibility index (CI) and Hausner ratio (HR) are determine by calculating bulk and tapped densities to provide a measure of the flow properties and compressibility of powders.

$$\text{Carr's compressibility index} = \frac{\text{Tapped density} - \text{Bulk density}}{\text{Tapped density}} \times 100$$

$$\text{Hausner's ratio} = \frac{\text{Tapped density}}{\text{Bulk density}}$$

Table 1.6 depicts the relationship between angle of repose, Carr's index and Hausner's ratio on the flow property of the power.

TABLE 1.6

Flowability scale

Flow	Angle of repose	Carr's index (%)	Hausner ratio
Excellent	25-30	5-10	1.0-1.11
Good	31-35	11-15	1.12-1.18
Fair to passable	36-40	16-20	1.19-1.25
Passable	41-45	21-25	1.26-1.34
Poor	46-55	26-31	1.35-1.45
Very Poor	>56	>32	> 1.46

Recently powder rheometers are also used to measure powder flow. Powder flow properties can be determined by measurements of bulk density and angle of repose.

1.5.4.2 Solubility Analysis

Solubility can be defined as the molarity of the substance in a solution that is in chemical equilibrium with an excess of the undissolved substance. The solubility is an important physicochemical property as it affects the dissolution parameters, rate of drug release, bioavailability of the drug and ultimately therapeutic efficiency. An important goal of the preformulation is to develop a method for making drug in its solution form. The solubility of the molecules in various solvents is determined as a first step. Solubility is usually determined in variety of commonly used solvents and some oils, if they are lipophilic. Solvents commonly used for solubility determination are water, buffers at various pH, methanol, isopropyl alcohol, ethyl alcohol, benzyl alcohol, castor oil, peanut oil, sesame oil. For therapeutic efficacy a drug must possess aqueous solubility in physiological pH range of 1 to 8 at 37 °C. Poor solubility of drug substance results in bioavailability problems.

(a) *Intrinsic Solubility*: It is the equilibrium solubility of the free acid or free base form of an ionisable compound at a pH where it is fully unionized. The increase in solubility of weakly basic/acidic drug in respective solution is due to intrinsic solubility. An increase in solubility in acidic aqueous solution compared to that in pure water, suggests weak base. An increase in solubility in alkaline solutions suggests weakly acid drug. The solubility of weakly acidic and basic drug as a function of pH can be predicted with the help of equation.

$$S = So \; \{1 + (K_1 / [H+])\} \quad \text{for weak acids}$$

$$S = So \; \{1 + ([H+] / K_2)\} \quad \text{for weak bases}$$

where, S = Solubility at given pH

S_o = Solubility of the unionized form

K_1 = Acid Dissociation constant

K_2 = Dissociation constant of conjugated acid

Methods to determine solubility

1. Equilibrium solubility method.
2. Turbidometric solubility method.
3. Nephlometric solubility method.
4. Ultrafiltration LC/MS solubility method.
5. Direct solubility method.

(b) *Ionization Constant (pK_a):* When we administer either a weakly basic or acidic drug, it will undergo ionization in GI fluids. Determination of the dissociation constant for a drug capable of ionization within a pH rang of 1 to 10 is important since solubility and consequently absorption, can be altered by orders of magnitude with changing pH. The relative conc. of unionized & ionized form of weakly acidic or basic drug in a solution at a given pH can be calculated using the Henderson-Hassel batch equation:-

pH = pK_a + log [unionized form] / [ionized form]   for weak bases

pH = pK_a + log [ionized form] / [unionized form]   for weak acids

The unionized forms are more lipid soluble & more rapidly absorbed from GIT.

Methods to determine pK_a

1. Potentiometric method.
2. Conductivity method.
3. Dissolution rate method.
4. Liquid-Liquid partition method.
5. Spectrophotometric method.

(c) *Partition Coefficient:* Partition Coefficient (oil/water) ($P_{o/w}$) is a measure of a drug's lipophilicity and is an indication of its ability to cross cell membranes. It is defined as the ratio of a unionized drug distributed between the organic and aqueous phases at equilibrium.

$$P_{o/w} = (C_{oil} / C_{water}) \text{ equilibrium}$$

C_{oil} – Concentration of oil

C_{water} – Concentration of water

The gastrointestinal membranes are primarily lipoidal in character hence the lipid solubility of a drug is an important factor in the assessment for its absorption. Partition coefficient provides a means of characterizing the lipophilic and hydrophilic nature of the drug which affects the rate and extent of drug absorption. Since biological membranes are lipoidal in nature. The rate of drug transfer for passively absorbed drugs is directly related to the lipophilicity of the molecule. The partition coefficient is commonly determined using an oil phase of octanol or chloroform in water.

Methods to determine partition coefficient

1. Shake Flask Method.
2. Chromatographic Method (TLC, HPLC).
3. Counter Current & Filter Probe method.

Applications of partition coefficient

- Measure of lipophilic/ hydrophilic character of molecules.
- Recovery of antibiotics from fermentation broth.
- Extraction of drug from biological fluid for therapeutic monitoring.
- Absorption of drug from dosage forms. (Ointments, Suppositories and Transdermal patches).
- Study of distribution of flavoring oil between oil & water in emulsion.

(d) ***Dissolution study***: In many instances dissolution rate or the time, it takes for the drug to dissolve in the fluid at the absorption site is the rate limiting step in the absorption process (drugs administered orally in solid forms such as tablets, capsules, or suspensions, and for those administered intramuscularly). Chemical form, crystal habit, particle size, surface area, wetting and solubility are the properties that widely influence the dissolution of the drug. Dissolution rate of drug can effect onset and intensity of action and control the overall bioavailability of drug form.

Dissolution rate of the drug substance as represented by modified Noyes-Whitney equation is given as follows (where surface area remains constant during disintegration).

$$\frac{dC}{dt} = \frac{DA}{hV}\left(C_s - C\right)$$

where,   D = diffusion coefficient in the dissolution medium

        h = thickness

        A = surface area

        V = volume

        C_s = concentration of the drug in saturated solution

        C = concentration at particular time t

Method to determine dissolution

1. ***Rotating disk method*:** This method allows for the determination of dissolution from constant surface area, obtained by compressing powder into a disc of known area with a die-punch apparatus.

2. ***Particulate dissolution*:** This method determines the dissolution of solids at different surface area. A weighed amount of powder sample from a particular sieve fraction is introduced in the dissolution medium. A constant speed propeller usually provides agitation. It is used to study the influence on dissolution of particle size, surface area & mixing with excipients.

(e) ***Common Ion Effect*:** A common ion significantly reduces, the solubility of a slightly soluble electrolyte. The "salting out" results from the removal of water molecules as solvent due to the competing hydration of other ions. So weakly basic drug which are given as HCl salts have decreased solubility in acidic solution. Eg. Chlortetracycline, Papaverine, Bromhexine, Triamterene, etc. The reverse process "salting in" arises with larger anions. (E.g. Benzoate, Salicylate) which can open the water structure. These hydrotropes increase the solubility of poorly water soluble compounds.

Methods to determine common ion effect

To identify a common ion interaction the IDR (Intrinsic dissolution rate) of HCl salt should be compared between

1. Water & water containing 1.2% W/V NaCl.
2. 0.05 M HCl & 0.9% NaCl in 0.05 M HCl.

Both saline media contains 0.2 M Cl⁻ which is typically encountered in fluids *in vivo*.

1.5.4.3 Stability Studies

Stability is defined as the extent to which a drug product maintains same properties and attribute within specified limits and throughout its shelf life which it possess at the time of manufacturing. Every drug substance possesses inherent stability, a critical factor in preformulation studies and plays a pivotal role in the development of the drug product. Various processing stages such as milling, drying, compression, storage condition, and gastrointestinal condition, influence the stability of a drug substance.

The first qualitative assessment in preformulation stability studies is chemical stability of a new drug, which includes both solid and solution state stability carried out under various condition for the administration, handling, compounding, storage and stability in presence of additives. Factors which influence chemical stability in development of dosage form design include temperature, pH and dosage form. A typical preformulation practice involves evaluating physical, chemical and compatibility stability. Stability studies help to select processing conditions, environmental condition and packaging system. Instability of drug may lead to undesired change in physical appearance, solubility, dissolution and ultimately bioavailability. Chemical degradation of drug may lead to a substantial loss of potency or formation of degraded product which may be unsafe or toxic.

(a) *Solid state stability*

Solid state reactions are much commlex, slower and more difficult to interpret than solution state reactions because of lesser molecular contacts between molecules of drug and excipient and also because of multiple phase transition (solid may convert to solid/ liquid/gas).

Many "solid state" reactions occur in solution. Major source of the solvent in solid phase are, residual moisture or drug or excipients, moisture in the capsule shell, melt of the drug / excipient , solvate or hydrate that loses its lattice solvent with time and temperature change.

Solid unstability basically results from hydrolysis, oxidation, photolysis and pyrolysis depending on the chemical structure of drug substances. Amorphous materials are less stable than their crystalline forms. Solid state stability generally comprises effect of temperature, humidity conditions, light and oxygen.

Techniques for solid state stability studies

- ✓ Solid State NMR Spectroscopy. (SSNMR)
- ✓ Powder X-ray diffraction. (PXRD)
- ✓ Fourier Transform IR. (FTIR)
- ✓ Raman Spectroscopy.
- ✓ Differential Scanning Calorimetry. (DSC).
- ✓ Thermo gravimetric Analysis. (TGA).

(b) *Solution phase stability*

Solution state stability is a critical part of the drug development process. The rate of degradation in solution form is rapid as than the dry solids. Stability studies of solution phase provides essential information for the development of efficacious product, helps in dosage form selection, in designing of dosage form and analytical method development. These studies include the effects of pH, temperature, light, oxygen,cosolvent and ionic Strength.

Degradation Pathways

Oxidation

It is a very common pathway for drug degradation in liquid and solid form. Oxidation occurs in two ways as, auto oxidation and by Free radical chain process. Functional groups having high susceptibility towards oxidation are alkenes, ethers, thioethers, Amines etc.

Factors affecting oxidation process:

- Oxygen
- Light.
- Heavy metals (Eg. Copper, iron, nickel, cobalt).
- Hydrogen & Hydroxyl ion.
- Temperature.

Oxidation can be Prevented by Reducing oxygen content, by storing the formulation in a tight closure/ containers or by addition of an antioxidant/ reducing agent /chain inhibitors.

There are various factors affecting stability of drug as depicted in figure 1.2.

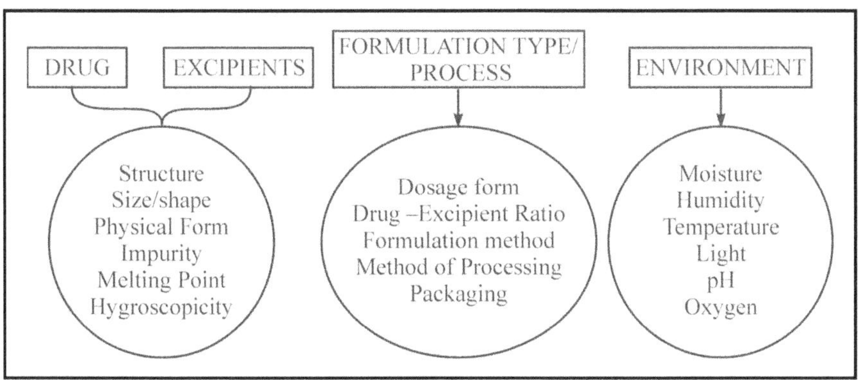

FIGURE 1.2 Factor affecting drug Stability.

Hydrolysis

It involves nucleophilic attack of labile groups. When the attack is by the solvent other than water, then it is known as solvolysis. Conditions that catalyze the breakdown are Presence of hydroxyl ion, hydride ion, divalent ion and heat and light. Hydrolysis can be prevented by adjusting the pH.

Photolysis

Electronic configuration of drug overlaps with the spectrum of sunlight or any artificial light where energy is absorbed by the electron resulting in excitation. As they are unstable, they release the acquired energy and return to the ground state by decomposing the drug. The phenomenon where molecules or excipients which absorb energy but do not participate themselves directly in the reaction but transfer the energy to others which cause cellular damage by inducing radical formation is known as photosensitization. Photo-decomposition can be prevented by proper packing, antioxidant, protecting from light, and use of photostabilizer.

Pathways of Photolysis:

- N-dealkylation - Dipenhydramine, Chloroquine,
- Dehalogenation - Furesemide
- Decarboxylation - Naproxen,
- Oxidation - Chlorpromazine
- Isomerization - Doxapine

Racemization

The interconversion from one isomer to another leads to different Pharmacokinetic, and pharmacological properties.e.g. Pilocarpine

L-epinephrine is 15 to 20 times more active than D-form, while activity of racemic mixture is half of the L-form.

Polymerization

It is a continuous reaction between molecules. More than one monomer reacts to form a polymer.

Eg. Darkening of glucose solution is attributed to polymerization of breakdown product [5- (hydroxyl methyl) furfural

Isomerization

It is the process involving change of one structure to another having same empirical formula but different properties in one or more respects.e.g. Tetracycline, Amphotericin B.(Trans-cis Isomerization)

Factors affecting drug stability

***pH*:** pH stability studies both in solution state and solid state, are performed to understand the behavior of drug substance with vehicles and in gastrointestinal environment. The acidity or the alkalinity of a solution influence the decomposition of most of the drug. Aspirin buffered solution, decomposes maximum above 10 pH and was found to be stable at pH 2.4. pH can also influence the rate of oxidation. pH decomposition profile of a drug is important in pre-formulation study to formulate the solution at a pH which is physiologically effective and stable.

***Elevated temperature studies*:** High temperature accelerates various reactions such as, oxidation, reduction and hydrolysis which lead to drug degradation. The elevated temperatures commonly used are 40, 50, and 60°C with ambient humidity. The samples stored at highest temperature are observed weekly for physical and chemical changes and compared to an appropriate control. If a substantial change is seen, samples stored at lower temperature are examined. If no changes are seen after 30 days at 60 degrees centigrade, the stability prognosis is excellent. All the drug products are stored at suitable temperatures to avoid thermal acceleration of decomposition.

***Stability under high humidity conditions*:** Water catalyses chemical reactions such as oxidation, hydrolysis and reduction reaction. Water promotes microbial growth. Solid drug samples can be exposed to different relative humidity conditions by keeping them in laboratory desiccators containing saturated solutions of various salts. The closed desiccators inturn are kept in oven to provide constant temperature. The pre-formulation data of this nature are useful in determining if the material should be protected and stored in controlled low humidity environment or if non aqueous solvent be used during formulation. Packing materials are chosen (usually glass and plastic) to prevent exposure of drug products to high humid condition.

The most common routes for the degradation of drugs are solvolysis, hydrolysis, photolysis, oxidation and racemization.

Photolytic stability: Light especially ultraviolet light enhances photolysis and humidity enhances hydrolytic decomposition. Photolysis affects drug stability through its energy or thermal effect which lead to oxidation. Many drugs fade or change their colour on exposure to light. Though the extent of degradations is small and limited to the exposed surface area, it presents aesthetic problem. Exposure of drug to 400 and 900 foot-candles of illumination for 4 and 2 week periods respectively is adequate to provide some idea on photosensitivity. Resulting data may be useful in determining if an amber coloured container is required or if colour masking dye should be used in the formulation. All the drug products are stored at suitable temperatures to avoid thermal acceleration of decomposition. Light sensitive materials are stored in amber coloured bottles.

Stability upon oxidation: Drug's sensitivity to oxidation can be examined by exposing it to atmosphere of high oxygen tension. Usually a 40% oxygen atmosphere allows for rapid evaluation. Samples are kept in desiccators equipped with three-way stop cocks, which are alternatively evacuated and flooded with desired atmosphere. The process is repeated 3 or 4 times to ensure 100% desired atmosphere. Results may be useful in predicting if an antioxidant is required in the formulation or if the final product should be packaged under inert atmospheric conditions. Proper packing keeping the oxygen content of the solution less and leaving very little head space in the bottle above the drug products are methods to fight against oxidation.

(c) ***Compatibility studies***: The knowledge of drug excipients interaction is useful for the formulation to select appropriate excipients. The described preformulation screening of drug excipients interaction requires only 5 mg of drug in a 50% mixture with the excipients to maximize the likelihood of obscuring an interaction. Mixtures should be examined under nitrogen to ultimate oxidation and paralytic effect at a standard heating rate on

DSC, over a temperature range, which will encompass any thermal changes due to both the drug and appearance or disappearance of one or more peaks in thermograms of drug excipient mixtures are considered as indication of interaction.

1.6   Methods for Characterizing Pharmaceutical Solids

Thermal methods

- Differential Scanning Calorimetry (DSC)
- Differential Thermal analysis (DTA)
- Thermogravimetric Analysis (TGA)
- Hot stage microscopy

Solubility methods

- Solubility
- Dissolution rate

Diffraction methods

- Single-crystal X-ray diffraction
- Powder X-ray diffraction
- Neutron diffraction

Spectroscopic methods

- UV spectroscopy
- Infrared spectroscopy
- Raman spectroscopy
- Solid-state NMR spectroscopy
- *Thermal methods*

  Thermal methods have wide application in the field of solid state analysis, detection of Crystallinity, polymorphism, impurity, moisture content, Characterization of hydrates/ solvates and study of drug - excipient and incompatability.

- *Differential Thermal analysis* **(DTA)**

  In this technique temperature difference between a substance & a reference material is measured as a function of temperature or time.   Difference in temperature i.e. Differential temp (Δt) is plotted against temp or a function of time.   Physical changes usually result in endothermic peak, whereas chemical reactions those of an oxidative nature are exothermic.

- ***Differential Scanning Calorimetry* (DSC)**

  DSC measures the temperature difference between the sample and a reference as a function of temperature or time when heating at a constant rate. DSC is similar to DTA except that the instrument measures the amount of energy required to keep the sample at the same temperature as the reference i.e. it measures the enthalpy of transition. Depending on the type of change within the sample, the thermal event may be endothermic or exothermic.

  If sample absorbs some amount of heat during phase transition then reaction is said to be endothermic. E.g. melting, sublimation, vaporization, desolvation. If sample released some amount of heat during phase transition, then reaction is said to be exothermic. E.g crystallization, polymerization.

- ***Thermo Gravimetric Analysis* (TGA)**

  Thermogravimetric methods are limited to decomposition & oxidation reaction and to such physical process like vaporization, sublimation, desorption. Thermal analytical system can be used for detection of impurities in pharmaceutical ingredient by recording TG Thermogram. This curves could be then be compared with the curve of reference standard.

- ***Hot stage microscopy* (HSM)**

  Drug crystals show thermal changes during the heating that can be examined under a microscope. Properties which are analyzed under a microscope include melting point, range of melting, crystal nucleation, crystal growth and crystal transformations. This technique is a simple and economical as it comprises of a heating stage with a sample holder and gaseous atmosphere control coupled with a suitable polarized-light microscope and a system that allows the capturing and measurements of observations and temperatures.

- ***X-ray diffraction***

  All diffraction methods are based on generation of X-rays. In an X-ray tube, which are directed at the sample, and the diffracted rays are collected and order of this diffraction is measured in form of graph. A key component of all diffraction is the angle between the incident and diffracted rays.

Single-crystal X-ray Diffraction is a non destructive analytical technique which provides detailed information about the internal lattice of crystalline substances such as, cell dimensions, bond lengths and angles.

X-ray powder Diffractometry is an analytical method to characterize crystalline material. X-ray diffraction is based on constructive interference of monochromatic X-rays and a crystalline sample. When X-rays interact with a solid material, the scattered beams can add together in a few directions and yield diffraction. The interaction of incident rays with the sample produces constructive interference when conditions satisfy Bragg's law.

$$\mathbf{n\ \lambda = 2\ d\ sin\theta}$$

Where,   n = order of diffraction

d = interatomic distance

θ = angle of incidence

Diffraction occur as a result of the interaction of radiation with electron of atom. When Bragg's condition is fulfilled, a peak is detected.

Application: determination of structure as, each drug has a unique XRD pattern that makes their identification possible,   detection of Impurity, Characterization of crystalline material and Polymorphism, study of phase transitions.

UV spectroscopy: The first requirement of any preformulation study is the development of a simple analytical method for quantitative estimation. Most of drugs have aromatic rings and/or double bonds as part of their structure and absorb light in UV range, UV spectroscopy being a fairly accurate and simple method is a performed estimation technique at early preformulation stages.

The absorption co-efficient of the drug can be determined by the formula:

$$E = \frac{AF}{X}$$

where,   A = Absorbance

F = dilution factor

X = weight of drug (mg)

It is now possible to determine concentration of drug in any solution by measuring absorbance.

C = AF / E mg / m*l*

Fourier Transforms Infrared Spectroscopy (FTIR)

FTIR spectroscopy is used extensively in pharmaceutical analysis for identification of structure and fingerprint identification. When IR radiation is passed through a sample, some radiation is absorbed by the sample and some transmitted. The resulting signal at the detector is a spectrum representing a molecular 'fingerprint' of the sample. The usefulness of infrared spectroscopy arises because different chemical structures produce different spectral fingerprints.

In preformulation FTIR is useful in study of polymorphism of solid crystals. Polymorphs show different IR characteristics which can be use as a tool for fingerprint identification.

Raman Spectroscopy

Raman spectroscopy is a nondestructive technique use for the characterization of polymorphism in solids and structure elucidation and functional group analysis. In this method sample is irradiated with monochromatic laser radiation, and the inelastic scattering of the source energy is used to obtain a vibrational spectrum of the analyte.

NMR / Solid-state NMR Spectroscopy (SSNMR)

NMR spectroscopy is non destructive techniques used to obtain physical, chemical, electronic and structural information about molecules. NMR involves the absorption of electromagnetic radiation in the radio-frequency of a longer wavelength spectrum.

The nuclei shift from lowest energy to a high energy orientation at a particular frequency. A plot of frequency versus intensity of radiation results in the NMR spectrum of a material. SSNMR spectroscopy is a kind of nuclear magnetic resonance (NMR) spectroscopy, characterized by the presence of anisotropic (directionally dependent) interactions. SSNMR is useful in identification of different crystalline forms of a compound

The major application of broadline NMR is in the measurement of the internuclear distances and other crystal parameters important in the study of polymorphism as well as hydrates and solvates. In addition to qualitative investigation of polymorphs and solvates, the quantitative measurement of polymorphs is also possible.

2 Tablets

2.1 Introduction

Drugs are prepared in various forms for administration and amongst other dosage forms, the solid form is most common and popular due to various advantages such as, accuracy of dosing, high patient compliance, stability, reproducibility and ease of production.

A tablet is a solid, hard, compressed, unit dosage form which encompasses a blend of one or more active substances and excipients. It offers safe and expedient way of administration of drug with accurate dosing and excellent stability. Tablets may differ greatly in size (round, triangle, oval or square shape) and weight depending on the dose of drug and the probable method of administration. Mostly, tablets are intended to be swallowed whole (oral), but some may be dissolved in the mouth (orodispersible), chewed (chewable), or dissolved in liquid before administration (Dispersible), and some may be placed in oral (sublingual/ buccal) and body cavity (rectal or intravaginal).

2.2 Advantages and Disadvantages of Tablets

2.2.1 Advantages

1. Easy and convenient to use.
2. Convenient in handling, packaging and transportation.
3. Accuracy of dose is maintained.
4. Physically and chemically stable.
5. Compactness and Portability.
6. Ease of administration, as no specialized person or technique is required.
7. Self administration is possible as compared with parenteral medication.

8. Easy product identification by means of different colour, shapes, size or embossing.

9. Tailor made release profile can be achieved. i.e., to release the drug at a particular site within the GIT to reduce degradation and side effects, to improve absorption at that site.

10. Tamper proof as compared with capsules

11. Least content variation.

2.2.2 Disadvantages

1. No dose flexibility.

2. Prompt termination of therapy is not possible

3. Difficult to prepare tablet with a high dose of drug into a tablet of suitable size.

4. Difficult to formulate with poorly compressible drug.

5. Difficult to formulate a drug with poor wettability.

6. Not preferable choice of medication in case of emergency.

7. Slow onset of action as compared to parenterals, liquid orals and capsules.

8. Difficult to swallow for kids, unconscious and geriatric patients.

2.3　Properties of Tablets

Tablets are available in many shape, but most popular are round, oval, oblong or capsule shape. An unusual shape of tablets is least popular with patients (difficult to swallow) and manufactures (chipping, packaging, and manufacturing problems). Tablets can be prepared in various shapes, sizes, surface marking depending on the types of punches and dies. Some tablets are in the shape of capsules, and are called as caplets. Tablets should be strong enough to resist the stress occuring during packaging, shipping and handling. The standards for tablet properties are given in most of the international pharmacopeias (USP/NF, EP, IP). Generally, tablet administered orally is most popular means of administering a drug; however, it can also be administered in other forms such as, implant, solution for vaginal, rectal and external use.

2.4   Types of Tablets

Different types of tablet formulations are available, which could be broadly classified based on various consideration as shown in Table 2.1.

TABLE 2.1

Classification of tablets

Mode of administration	
Tablets for ingestion	Tablets to be swallowed with water
	Chewable tablet
	Dispersible tablet
Tablets used in the oral cavity	Lozenges and troches
	Sublingual tablet
	Buccal tablet
	Dental cones
	Mouth dissolved tablet
Tablets instilled into body cavity	Rectal tablet
	Vaginal tablet
	Implants
	Ear cone
Tablets used to prepare solution	Effervescent tablet
	Hypodermic tablet
	Dispensing tablet
	Tablet triturate
According to drug release rate	
Immediate release tablet	Disintegrating tablet
	- Chewable tablet
	- Sublingual tablet
	- Buccal tablet
	- Effervescent tablet
Modified release tablet	Extended release tablet
	Delayed release tablet
According to method of manufacturing	
Tablets prepared by compression method	• Standard compressed tablets
	• Multiple compressed tablets
	I. Compression coated tablet
	II. Layered tablet
Tablets prepared by molding method	Tablet triturates
	Lozenges
On the basis of coating	
Uncoated tablets	Conventional tablets
Coated tablets	Sugar coated
	Film-coated tablet
	Modified release coated tablets
	Enteric coated tablets

2.4.1 On the Basis of Mode of Administration

2.4.1.1 Tablets for Ingestion

These types of tablets are designed to release the drug within the gastrointestinal tract for systemic or local effect. It is usually swallowed or dissolved in water before taking.

1. *Tablets to be swallowed with water*: It is most widely preferred form of medication. These tablets are meant to be swallowed intact along with water. These may again be classified on the basis of different methods of manufacturing and release behavior.

2. *Chewable tablets*: These are intended to be broken and chewed in between the teeth before ingestion. Antacid and vitamins tablets are usually prepared as chewable tablets. The advantage of this medication is that it can be taken at any time or when water is not available. For patients who have difficulty in swallowing such as children and geriatric, chewable tablet serves as an attractive alternative as mentioned in 2.4.1.1.

3. *Dispersible tablets*: These tablets disintegrate either rapidly in water, to form a stabilized suspension, or disperse instantaneously in the mouth to be swallowed without the aid of water. So, it's preferred for pediatric patients who cannot swallow a solid dosage form and the API is unstable if formulated in liquid formulation. This is also helpful for patients having prolonged illness who are prone to nausea sensations if they have to swallow a tablet.

2.4.1.2 Tablets used in the Oral Cavity

The tablets under this group are aimed to release drug in oral cavity to provide local action in this region at the site or to get fast systemic effect. The tablets under this category avoids first-pass metabolism, decomposition of drug in gastric environment and gives rapid onset of action.

1. *Lozenges and troches*: These tablets are flat faced with at least about 18 mm in diameter and dissolve in the mouth to obtain continuous effect on the mucous membrane of the throat or they are intended to be placed in the mouth or pharynx. The compressed tablet is called troches and the tablets produced by fusion or candy molding process are called lozenges. The tablet generally contains sucrose or lactose and gelatin solution to impart smooth taste. Drugs usually given in the form of Lozenges for local action in

mouth throat are: antiseptics, antibiotics, demulcents, antitussive agents or astringents.

2. ***Sublingual tablets*:** They are to be placed under the tongue that produces immediate systemic effect by enabling the drug absorption directly from mucosal lining of the mouth beneath the tongue. The absorbed drug goes to mesenteric circulation, which connects to stomach via portal vein. Thus, absorption through oral cavity avoids first-pass metabolism.

3. ***Buccal tablets*:** Buccal tablets are placed in the buccal pouch where they dissolve or disintegrate slowly and absorbed through oral mucosa without passing into the alimentary tract.

4. ***Dental cones*:** These tablets are designed to be placed in the empty socket remaining after a tooth extraction. Main purpose behind the use of these types of tablets is either to prevent multiplication of bacteria in the socket by employing a slow releasing antibacterial compound or to reduce bleeding by an astringent or coagulant containing tablet. It is formulated to dissolve or erode slowly in presence of a small volume of serum or fluid over 20-30 minute's period.

5. ***Chewable tablets*:** As mentioned in 2.4.1.1.

2.4.1.3 Tablets Administered by other Routes

These tablets are administered by route other than the oral cavity and so the drugs are prevented from passing through gastro intestinal tract. These tablets may be inserted into other body cavities or directly placed below the skin to be absorbed into systemic circulation from the site of application.

1. ***Vaginal tablets*:** Vaginal tablet are designed to undergo slow dissolution and drug release in vaginal cavity. The shape is kept ovoid or pear shaped to facilitate retention in vagina. These tablets generally contain the drugs such as antibacterial, antiseptics or astringents to treat vaginal infections or release steroids for systemic absorption *e.g*: Estradiol vaginal tablets, Clotrima-zole vaginal tablets etc., would be nice if given example for all types.

2. ***Rectal tablets*:** Rectal tablet are designed to undergo slow dissolution and drug release in rectal cavity.

3. *Implantable tablets*: Implants or depot tablets are inserted into subcutaneous tissue by surgical procedures where they are very slowly absorbed over a period of a month or a year. A special injector with a hollow needle and plunger is used to administer the rod shaped tablet or any other shape. The tablets may be pellet, cylindrical or rosette shaped with diameter not more than 8 mm. Implant pellets are generally used for the administration of hormones.

2.4.1.4 Tablets used to Prepare Solution

The tablets under this category are required to be dissolved first in water or other suitable solvents before administration or application. This solution may be used for ingestion, parenteral application or for topical use depending upon type of medicament used.

1. *Effervescent tablets*: Effervescent tablets are designed to break down rapidly with the simultaneous release of carbon dioxide. These tablets are prepared by compressing the drug with mixtures of organic acid and carbonate source to form potassium, sodium, calcium or magnesium salts of the acid and buffers the solution to a normal pH. One of the biggest advantages is that they deliver drugs to the body rapidly, because the drug is delivered in the form of a solution, which is easy to absorb. This preparation makes the tablet palatable. Disadvantage of effervescent tablet is the difficulty of producing a chemically stable product.

2. *Hypodermic tablets*: These tablets contain one or more readily water soluble ingredients and are intended to be added to the sterile water or water for injection to form a clear solution which is to be injected parenterally.

3. *Dispensing tablets*: These tablets dissolve completely in liquid to produce solution of definite concentration. Water soluble tablets are intended for application after dissolution in water. Antibiotics and certain vitamins are given in the form of mouth wash, gargle, skin lotion, douche etc. Mouth wash, gargle, skin lotion, douche antibiotic, certain vitamins are given in this type of formulations.

4. *Tablet triturates*: These are small cylindrical, molded or compressed disc of varying size, containing a diluent usually consisting of dextrose (glucose) or a mixture of lactose and powdered sucrose and also a moistening agent or excipients, such as dilute alcohol.

2.4.2 According to Drug Release Rate

2.4.2.1 Immediate Release Tablet

This type of tablet is intended to release immediately after administration. These are designed to release the drug immediately or atleast as quickly as possible after administration. This is useful if a fast onset of action is required for therapeutic reasons. It is the most common type like disintegrating tablet, chewable tablet, sublingual tablet (which are explained before) buccal tablet and effervescent tablet.

2.4.2.2 Modified Release Tablet

Modified-released tablet is either uncoated or coated. The drug release only occurs some time after the administration or for a prolonged period of time or to a specific target in the body. This contains special additives or prepared by special procedure which separately or together is intended to modify the rate of release of the drug into the gastrointestinal tract. It prolongs the effect of drug and also reduces the frequency of administration of drug.

1. *Delayed action tablets*: These tablets are intended to release drug after some specified time of administration in order to protect the drug from degradation in the low pH environment of the stomach or to protect the stomach from irritation by the drug. In these cases, drug release should be delayed until the dosage form has reached the small intestine.

2. *Enteric-coated tablets*: Enteric-coated tablets are coated with materials that prevent the release of drug in stomach whereas releases it after reaching the upper part of intestine. It delays release of the medication until after it leaves the stomach.

3. *Sustained release/controlled release tablets*: These types of dosage form are designed to achieve a prolonged therapeutic effect by continuously releasing medication over an extended period of time after administration of the single dose. These systems maintain the rate of drug release over a prolonged period.

2.4.3 According to Method of Manufacturing

2.4.3.1 Tablets Prepared by Compression Method

These types of tablets are obtained by compressing uniform volume of particles using tablet compression machine.

A. Standard compressed tablets

These are uncoated tablets made by compression provide rapid disintegration and drug release for local action in gastro-intestinal tract or systemic action.

B. Multiple compressed tablets

Multiple compressed tablets are prepared by subjecting the fill materials to more than a single compression.

(a) *Compression coated tablet*: In this system the entire surface of inner core is completely surrounded by the outer coat. The technique is simple and used to provide tablet with adjustable drug release which depends on the composition of core and coat layer. It can be used to deliver one or more drugs.

(b) *Layered tablet*: These are prepared by initial compaction of a portion of fill material in the die followed by additional fill material and compression to form multilayered tablet. Each layer may contain a different drug. Layered tablets are prepared due to the incompatibility between the two drugs or to alter the drug release from different layers.

C. Tablets prepared by molding method

These type of tablets are obtained using tablet mold. It is restricted for small-dose tablet and small-scale production. *e.g.* Tablet triturates, Lozenges.

2.4.4 On the Basis of Coating

A. Uncoated Tablets: Conventional Tablets

B. Coated Tablets

(a) *Sugar coated tablets*: The tablet that contains active ingredient(s) of unpleasant taste are covered with sugar coating to make it more palatable.

(b) *Film-coated tablets*: Film coating of tablets are carried out to protect the drug from atmospheric conditions and masks the objectionable taste and the odour of drug.

(c) *Modified release coated tablets*: They are intended to modify the rate of release of the drug into the gastrointestinal tract by using polymers to sustain the release of drug for a predetermined period of time. It prolongs the effect of drug, improves bioavailability and also reduces the frequency of administration of drug.

   (d) ***Enteric coated tablets***: Some drugs are prone to be destroyed by gastric juice or cause irritation to the stomach. This can be solved by coating the tablet with an enteric coating polymer (cellulose acetate phthalate). This polymer is insoluble in gastric contents but readily dissolves in intestinal contents. So there is delay in the disintegration of dosage form until it reaches the small intestine.

2.5   Tablet Manufacturing Methods

The manufacture of tablets is a complex multistage process where final dosage form is produced by transforming physical characteristics of drugs and excipients at every stage of processing. The tablet manufacturing process can be broadly classified as granulation (wet granulation or dry granulation) and direct compression methods. Various unit operations (Figure 2.1) such as particle size reduction, sieving, blending, granulation, drying, compaction and optional coating are involved in manufacturing of tablets.

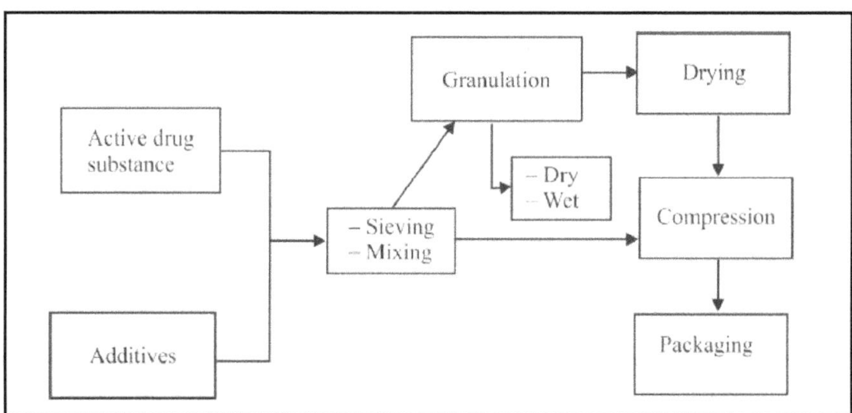

FIGURE 2.1 Basic process of tablet manufacturing.

Steps involved in the tablet manufacturing are shown in Table 2.2.

TABLE 2.2

Steps involved in different tablet manufacturing process

Wet granulation	Dry granulation	Direct compression
1. Milling and mixing of drugs and excipients	1. Milling and mixing of drugs and excipients	1. Milling and mixing of drugs and excipients
2. Preparation of binder Solution	2. Compression into slugs or roll compaction	2. Compression of tablet
3. Wetting the mass of drug massing by addition of binder solution or granulating solvent	3. Milling and screening of slugs and compacted powder into granules	
4. Screening of wet mass	4. Mixing with lubricant and disintegrant	
5. Drying of the wet Granules	5. Compression of tablet	
6. Screening of dry Granules		
7. Blending with lubricant and disintegrant to reduce the friction		
8. Compression of tablet		

2.5.1 Granulation Methods

Granulation is a size enlargement process of particle to produce larger multi particulate spherical entities called as granules for improving flow and compressibility.

Rationale for Granulation

Important aspects in the process of granulation are:

- Improve flow,
- Improve content uniformity,
- Improve compression characteristics,
- Decrease dust generation,
- Reduce cross contamination of drug product Improve the appearance of the tablet.

Granulation can be achieved by the use of binder solution (wet granulation) or dry binder (dry granulation). Wet granulation is often chosen over dry granulation because of dust elimination, single pot processing, uniformity of API (Active pharmaceutical ingredient) content (low dose API) and obtaining predictable granulation end point determination. Examples of wet granulation methods include fluid bed, high shear, palletization techniques, such as extrusion spheronization, spray drying, etc. The quality of this solid oral dosage form is as a general rule, primarily governed by the physicochemical properties of the powder/granulation from which the tablets are composed. Dry granulation (roll compaction or slugging) involves the compaction of powders at high pressures into large, often poorly formed tablets or compacts. These compacts are then milled and screened to form a granulation of the desired particle size. The advantage of dry granulation is the elimination of heat and moisture in the processing. Dry granulations can be produced by extruding powders between hydraulically operated rollers to produce thin cakes that are subsequently screened or milled to give the desired granule size.

***Granules are prepared by two methods*:**

1. Wet granulation
2. Dry granulation
   (a) Slugging
   (b) Roller compaction

2.5.1.1 Wet Granulation

Wet granulation process simply involves wet massing of the powder particles with a granulating fluid (aqueous or non-aqueous), wet sizing and drying. The fluid contains a solvent, which must be volatile so that it can be removed by drying and be non-toxic. Typical liquids include water, ethanol and isopropanol, either alone or in combination. Wet granulation is often chosen over dry granulation because of several advantages.

Advantages

- Elimination of dust
- Prevents segregation of powders
- Better drug content uniformity
- It improves flow properties and compression characteristics and increases density of granules

Disadvantages

- Multiple processing steps
- Expensive process since more laborious, time, equipment and space requirements
- Loss of material during various stages of processing
- Not suitable for moisture sensitive or thermolabile drugs
- Over wetting of granules can leads to large size lumps formation.

Special Wet Granulation Techniques

(i) ***High shear mixture granulation***: High shear mixture has been widely used for blending and granulation, which is accompanied by high mechanical agitation by an impeller and a chopper. Mixing densification and agglomeration are achieved through shear and compaction force exerted by the impeller.

Advantages

- Short processing time
- Less amount of liquid binders required
- Highly cohesive material can be granulated.

Disadvantages

- Mechanical degradation of fragile particles
- chemical degradation of thermolabile material
- Over wetting of granules, can lead to large size lumps formation.

(ii) ***Fluid bed granulation***: Fluid bed granulation is a process by which granules are produced in single equipment by spraying a binder solution onto a fluidized powder bed. The material processed by fluid bed granulation are finer, free flowing and homogeneous.

Advantages

- It reduces dust formation during processing thus avoiding cross contamination
- It reduces product loss
- It improves worker safety.

Disadvantages

- The fluid bed cleaning is labor-intensive and time consuming
- Difficulty of assuring reproducibility.

(iii) ***Extrusion-spheronization***: A multiple step process consists of wet mixing, extrusion, spheronization and drying is helpful in making uniform sized spherical particles.

Advantages

- Ability to incorporate higher levels of active components without producing excessively larger particles
- Applicable to both immediate and controlled release dosage form.

Disadvantages

- The process is laborious and exhaustive
- Time consuming.

(iv) ***Spray drying***: It is a unique granulation technique in which a dry granular product is made from a solution or a suspension. It involves, atomization of a liquid feed into fine droplets, mixing of these sprayed droplets with a heated gas stream, allowing the liquid to evaporate and leave dried solids and separation of the dried powder from the gas stream.

Advantages

- Rapid and continuous process
- Reduces overall cost by avoiding intensive drying and granulation steps
- Minimal exposure to dust
- Suitable for heat sensitive product.

Disadvantages

1. More labour and time consuming
2. Thermal efficiency is relatively low.

2.5.1.2 Dry Granulation

Dry granulation involves processing steps of blending and compaction of the ingredients followed by milling and screening to form granules of the desired and uniform particle size. The advantage of dry granulation is the elimination of heat and moisture in the processing. This method is suitable for moisture and heat sensitive materials.

Two main dry granulation processes are:

(i) *Slugging process*: This process involves compression of dry powder into the dies of a large capacity tablet press and is compacted by means of flat faced punches. The compacted mass is called as slugs and the process is called as slugging. These slugs are converted to appropriate size granules by milling and screening for final compression into tablets.

(ii) *Roller compaction*: Dry granulations can be produced by extruding powders between two hydraulically operated rollers to produce thin cakes (strips) that are subsequently screened or milled to give the desired granule size.

2.5.1.3 Advancements in Granulation

(a) *Steam granulation*: It is modification of wet granulation method. Steam is used as a binder instead of water. It offers several advantages which include:

- Granules obtained from steam method are more spherical have large surface area hence produce increased dissolution rate of the drug when compared to granules

- Higher diffusion rate into powders

- More favorable thermal balance during drying step

- Shorter processing time

- Compared to the use of organic solvent water vapor is environmental friendly, thus no health hazards to operators

(b) *Melt granulation/Thermoplastic granulation*: Granulation is achieved by the addition of binder, which is in solid state at room temperature but melts at the higher temperatures. Melted binder such as poly ethylene glycol, stearic acid, cetyl or stearyl alcohol, and various waxes act like a binding liquid.

Advantages

- There is no need of drying phase since dried granules are obtained by cooling it to room temperature. Moreover, amount of liquid binder can be controlled precisely and the production and equipment costs are reduced

- It is useful for granulating water sensitive material and also suitable for preparing sustained release granules or solid dispersions.

Disadvantages

- Not suitable for thermo labile substances
- Non reproducible method

(c) ***Moisture activated dry granulation*****:** It involves minimal moisture addition to powder blend, distribution and agglomeration in the form of granules. No drying step is required. It produces granules with excellent flowability and uniformity, and is applicable to controlled release.

(d) ***Thermal adhesion granulation process*****:** This method is used for direct tableting formulations. Granules are prepared from mixtures of excipients having low moisture content or low content of pharmaceutically acceptable solvent. This method utilizes less water or solvent than traditional wet granulation method. It provides granules with good flow properties and binding capacity to form tablets of low friability, adequate hardness and have a high uptake capacity for active substances whose tableting is poor or difficult.

(e) ***Foam granulation*****:** In this method liquid binders are added as aqueous foam. It has several benefits over wet granulation such as

- No plugging problems
- No over wetting
- Less binder requirements
- No detrimental effects on granulate
- Useful for granulating water sensitive formulations
- Reduces drying time
- Uniform distribution of binder throughout the powder bed
- Reduce manufacturing time

2.5.1.4 Direct Compression

Direct compression is the simplest and most economical method for the manufacturing of tablets because it requires less processing steps than other techniques such as wet granulation and roller compaction. Direct compression avoids many of the problems associated with wet and dry granulations. Most pharmaceutically active ingredients cannot be compressed directly into tablets due to lack of flowability, cohesion properties and lubrication. Therefore, they must be blended with other directly compressible ingredients to manufacture satisfactory tablets.

Advantages

- Low labour input
- Less manufacturing cost
- Fewer processing steps hence, the validation and documentation requirements are reduced.
- Suitable for heat and moisture sensitive drugs.

Disadvantages

- Problems in the uniform distribution of low dose drugs
- Drugs having high dose, poor compressibility and flowability are not suitable
- Segregation of particles may occur due to the difference in particle size or density of drug and excipients
- The dry state of the material during mixing may induce static charge and lead to segregation.

Some of the most widely used direct compression fillers are:

- Di-Pac is a directly compressible, co-crystallized sugar consisting of 97% sucrose and 3% modified dextrin.
- Nu-Tab is a roller compacted granulated product consisting of sucrose, invert sugar, corn starch and magnesium stearate.
- Emdex is produced by hydrolysis of starch and consists of aggregates of dextrose microcrystals intermixed and cohered with a small quantity of higher molecular weight sugars.

Cellulose derivatives (Microcrystalline cellulose, Hydroxy propyl cellulose)

Saccharides (*e.g*: lactose and mannitol)

Mineral salts (*e.g*: dicalcium phosphate, calcium carbonate)

Partially pregelatinzed starch (Starch 1500®)

Modified Sucrose: (Di-Pac, Nu-Tab, Emdex)

Table 2.3 provides the advantages and limitations of different table manufacturing methods.

TABLE 2.3

Tablet manufacturing methods-advantages and limitations

Method	Advantages	Limitations
Direct compression	• Simple, economical process • No heat or moisture, so good for thermolabile and moisture sensitive drugs	• Not suitable for all API, • Segregation potential • Expensive excipients
Wet granulation	• Robust process suitable for most compound • Can reduce elasticity problems. • reduces segregation potential	• Expensive: time and energy consuming process • Stability issues for moisture sensitive and thermolabile drugs • Specialized equipments are required
Dry granulation	• Suitable for moisture sensitive and thermolabile drugs	• Expensive equipment. • Dusty procedure. • Not suitable for all drugs

2.6   Formulation of Tablets

Tablet dosage form is composed of two main ingredients: (1) Active pharmaceutical ingredients (API) or main drug and, (2) inactive ingredients also termed as additives or excipients. Selection of proper API and excipients plays a very important role in formulation development as it may affect performance of dosage form.

Dose of drug may have impact on various tablet properties. Low dose drug (Misoprostol, ramipril,) may have content uniformity problems due to non uniform distribution of drug in formulation. High dose drugs (Metformin, paracetamol) size of tablet is the critical issue. Solubility of API may influence the choice of manufacturing process as it might affect dissolution parameters. Particle size of drug may be important for solubility and dissolution. Low melting point drug (Nifedipine, gliclazide) may result in sticking problems or soft tablets during compression. pK_a of drug is important factor in solubility and absorption of the drug. Aspirin, meloxicam shows better solubility in basic pH. Bulk density flow property and compatibility of drug may affect hardness, content variation and weight variation. Moisture content and Hygroscopicity of drug leads to processing problems. Drugs sensitivity towards light, heat, moisture effect the stability of dosage form. Incompatibility between drugs and excipients is another important parameter to be considered as it may lead to degradation.

Pharmaceutical additives can be defined as any substance other than the active drug that has been appropriately evaluated for safety and is included to assist in formulation, improve stability, bioavailability or patient acceptability. These are also included to improve the organoleptic properties of formulations. The additives perform the following functions in manufacturing process:

1. Aid processing of the system during manufacture
2. Protect, support or enhance stability, bioavailability or patient acceptability
3. Assist in product identification
4. Enhance any other attribute of the overall safety and effectiveness of the drug product during storage or use.

Ideally all the excipients must be chemically inert, non-hygroscopic, compatible with drug, regulatory compliant, non-toxic, have acceptable taste and be inexpensive. The pharmaceutical industry uses many different types of excipients, which can be classified as primary excipients based on their functionality or as secondary excipients based on the way they are used. The criteria for the selection of excipients are as given in Figure 2.2.

2.6.1 Diluents

Diluents or bulking agents are inert substances used to make up the required bulk or volume when the dose of drug in a tablet is inadequate to produce tablets of adequate weight and size. Usually the range of diluents may vary from 5-80%. Diluents are also synonymously known as fillers. Diluents are often added to tablet formulations for secondary reasons like to provide better tablet properties such as:

- To provide improved cohesion
- To allow direct compression for manufacturing
- To enhance flow property
- To adjust weight of tablet as per die capacity

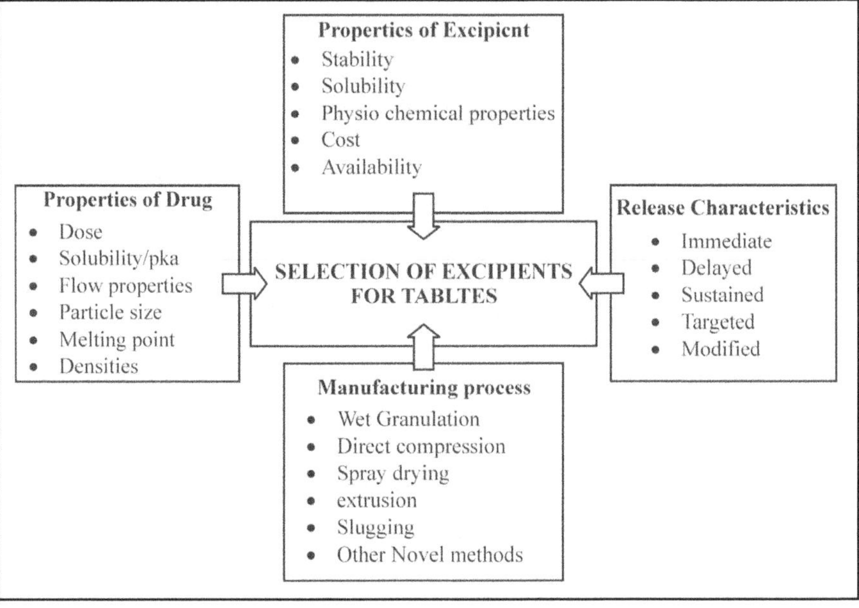

FIGURE 2.2 Criteria for excipients selection.

Diluents must meet certain basic criteria for satisfactory performance in tablet dosage form. They are as follows:

- It should not react and be compatible with the drug substance.
- It should not alter the functions of other excipients.
- It should not have any physiological or pharmacological activity of its own.
- It should have consistent physical and chemical characteristics.
- It should neither promote nor contribute to segregation of the granulation or powder blend to which they are added.

- It should neither support microbiological growth in the dosage form nor contribute to any microbiological load.

- It should neither adversely affect the dissolution of the product nor interfere with the bioavailability of active pharmaceutical ingredient.

2.6.1.1 Classification of Diluents

Tablet diluents or fillers can be divided into following categories:

(i) Organic materials – Carbohydrate and modified carbohydrates.

(ii) Inorganic materials – Calcium phosphates and others.

(iii) Co-processed Diluents– Emdex (93% dextrose and 7% maltodextrin), Cellactose (MCC and Lactose)

1. *Lactose monohydrate (hydrous)*: Lactose monohydrate is water soluble, not directly compressible and has poor flow properties. It produces hard tablet and hardness further increases on storage. It undergoes discolouration when formulated with amines and alkaline materials (i.e., browning or maillard reaction). It contains approximately 5% moisture and hence can be a potential source of instability especially with moisture sensitive drugs. It is inexpensive.

   (a) Lactose anhydrous: Lactose anhydrous is directly compressible inexpensive diluent. It does not exhibit free flowing property. It can pick up moisture at elevated humidity as a result of which, changes in tablet dimensions may occur. It does not undergo a maillard reaction which can lead to browning and discolouration of tablet surface.

   (b) Spray dried lactose: It is directly compressible diluent, which exhibits good free flowing characteristics. Its compressibility decreases when dried below 3% moisture level. It has high dilution potential. It is more prone to darkening in the presence of excess moisture, amines and other compounds due to the presence of a furaldehyde. Usually, neutral or acid lubricant should be used when spray dried lactose is employed. It is expensive compared to anhydrous and hydrous lactose.

2. *Sucrose*: It is water soluble and possesses good binding properties. It is slightly hygroscopic. It is inexpensive. It produces gritty

mouth feel (i.e., it is not free from grittiness). It is a calorie contributor and is cariogenic. Some of the sucrose based diluents have trade names as, Sugar Tab, Di pac, and Nu Tab.

3. *Mannitol*: Mannitol is an optical isomer of sorbitol. It exhibits poor flow properties, most expensive sugar and is water soluble. It is widely used in chewable tablets because of its negative heat of solution, its slow solubility and its mild cooling sensation in mouth. It can be used in vitamin formulation, where moisture sensitivity may create a problem. It is comparatively non hygroscopic. It is free from grittiness. It possesses low caloric value and is noncarcinogenic.

4. *Sorbitol*: It is highly compressible diluent and is water soluble. It is hygroscopic in nature. It has good mouth feel and sweet cooling taste. It is free from grittiness, possesses low caloric value and is noncarcinogenic. It is often combined with mannitol in formulations in order to reduce diluents cost.

5. *Microcrystalline cellulose*: Microcrystalline cellulose (Avicel) derived from a special grade of purified alpha wood cellulose by severe acid hydrolysis It is a direct compressible material available in two tablet grades: PH 101 (powder) and PH 102 (granules). It undergoes plastic deformation on compression and hence it is more sensitive to lubricants. It exhibits good flowability. It is water insoluble. It is relatively expensive material.

6. *Calcium phosphates*: The calcium phosphates include, the dihydrate and anhydrous form of dibasic calcium phosphate and tribasic calcium phosphate. They are widely used as wet granulation and direct compression diluents in tablet formulation. Bulk density of calcium phosphates is higher than that of organic fillers. Dibasic calcium phosphate is available commercially under the trade name Di-Tab and Emcompress. An anhydrous form of dibasic calcium phosphate is available commercially under the trade name A-Tab and Tribasic calcium phosphate is available under the trade name Tri-Tab.

These are directly compressible and are characterized by brittle fracture on compression during tablet process. Hard tablets are produced when calcium phosphates are used as diluents. They exhibit good flow properties, inexpensive and are non hygroscopic.

7. *Starch*: Starch is obtained from corn, wheat or potatoes has poor flow and compression properties and possesses moisture content

between 11 and 14%. Various directly compressible starches are sta-Rx 1500. Two hydrolyzed starches are Emdex and Celutab which is 90-92% dextrose and 3-5% maltose. They are free flowing and directly compressible.

2.6.2 Binders/Adhesives

Binders or adhesives are the substances that promote cohesiveness. It is utilized for converting powder into granules through a process known as granulation. Binders hold the materials in a tablet together to ensure required mechanical strength and hardness. Types of binders available and their properties are as shown in Table 2.3 and 2.4.

2.6.2.1 Classification of Binders

Binders can also be classified according to their application:

1. ***Solution binders*:** These are dissolved in a solvent such as water and alcohol *e.g.* starch gelatin, cellulose derivatives, polyvinyl pyrrolidone sucrose and polyethylene glycol.

2. ***Dry binders*:** These are added to the powder blend as part of a direct powder compression formula. *e.g*: cellulose derivatives, carbopol, methyl cellulose, polyvinyl pyrrolidone and polyethylene glycol.

TABLE 2.4

Classification of binders

Sugars	Sucrose, Liquid glucose, xylitol, sorbitol or maltitol
Natural binders	Acacia, Tragacanth, Gelatin, Starch Paste, Alginic Acid
Semisynthetic polymer	Methyl Cellulose, Ethyl Cellulose, Hydroxy propyl methyl cellulose (HPMC), Hydroxy Propyl Cellulose, Sodium Carboxy Methyl Cellulose,
Synthetic polymer	Polyvinyl Pyrrolidone (PVP), Polymethacrylates (Eudragits)

Characteristics of some commonly binders used with their advantages and disadvantages are as shown in Table 2.5.

TABLE 2.5

Characteristics of commonly used binder

Binders	Con. (%w/w)	Advantages	Limitations
Starch paste	5-25	Good binding ability.	Time consuming process, High variability in preparation of starch paste
Acacia/ Tragacanth	10-25	Good binding ability when used in liquid form	Variability in composition and performance
Pregelatinized starch	5 – 10	Cold water soluble, so easier to prepare can be used as binders in direct compression as well as Wet Granulation.	Only functions as a binder.
Polyvinyl pyrrolidone	1-5	Available in various ranges of molecular weight/ viscosities. Soluble in water and ethanol. The drug release is not altered on storage.	Upon storage prolonging the disintegration time and dissolution
Hydroxypropyl methyl cellulose	2 - 8	It is soluble in different solvent systems Used as a binder in either wet or dry granulation processes.	Produce hard granules, if binder concentration and kneading time is increased.
Methylcellulose	1 - 5	Various viscosity grades are available	Produce hard granules, if binder concentration and kneading time is increased.

2.6.3 Disintegrants

Disintegrants are included in the formulation to facilitate breaking up of tablet into small fragments when it comes in contact with liquid. Disintegrants expand, dissolve and release the drug when it comes in contact with fluid. They may function by promoting the penetration of water into the tablet by capillary action which leads to swelling and bursting of tablets (Deaggregation) which releases the drug particles and get dissolved in the gastric fluid from which the drug is absorbed.

All disintegrants are hygroscopic and hence draw liquid into the tablet ("liquid uptake" or "wicking action"). This may lead to the generation of hydrostatic pressure due to which they absorb the liquid and swell extensively (Sodium Starch Glycolate). Some disintegrants recover their shape with little swelling (Crospovidone) and some swell radially and straighten out (Croscarmellose Sodium).

A. **Starch:** Starch is used in the concentration of 5-20% of the tablet weight. The mechanism of action of starch is wicking and restoration of deformed starch particles on contact with aqueous fluid and in doing so release of certain amount of stress which is responsible for disruption of hydrogen bonding formed during compression.

   The concentration of starch used is of prime concern. If used below the optimum concentration it results in poor disintegration (insufficient channels for capillary action) and if it is used above optimum concentration then it will be difficult to compress the tablet.

B. Pregelatinized starch: Pregelatinized starch is produced by the hydrolyzing and rupturing of the starch grain. It is a directly compressible disintegrant and its optimum concentration is 5-10%. The main mechanism of action of pregelatinized starch is through swelling.

C. **Modified starch:** Starch is modified by carboxy methylation followed by cross linking to have a high swelling properties and faster disintegration. Low substituted carboxymethyl starches are available in the market as Explotab and Primogel. Mechanism of action of these modified starches are rapid and extensive swelling with minimum gelling. And its optimum concentration is 4-6 %. They are highly efficient at low concentration because of their greater swelling capacities.

D. **Ion-exchange resin:** Ion exchange resin (Ambrelite®IPR-88) has highest water uptake capacity than other disintegrating agents. Disadvantage is that it has tendency to adsorb certain drugs.

E. **Clays:** Clays such as veegum HV and bentonite have been used as disintigrants at 10% level.

F. **Miscellaneous:** This includes disintegrants like surfactants (Aerosol OT®), gas producing disintegrants (bicarbonates with citric acid). Gas producing disintegrating agents are used in soluble tablet, dispersible tablet and effervescent tablet.

2.6.4 Superdisintegrants

These are agents which increase the disintegration of tablets thereby reduced the disintegration time. They act by swelling which exerts pressure in the radial direction that causes tablet to burst and disintegrate. Swelling can also accelerate absorption of water leading to an enormous increase in the volume of granules to promote disintegration. Superdisintegrants show excellent disintegration activity at low concentrations. Major limitations of these superdisintegrants are relatively high cost and hygroscopic nature, which could negatively affect the stability of moisture sensitive API.

The types of superdisintigrants are shown in Table 2.6.

TABLE 2.6

Types of superdisintegrants

Superdisintegrants	Example
Crosslinked cellulose	Crosscarmellose, Ac-Di-Sol, Nymce ZSX Primellose, Solutab, Vivasol
Crosslinked PVP	Crosspovidone, Crosspovidon M, Kollidon Polyplasdone XL
Crosslinked starch	Sodium starch glycolate, Explotab, Primogel
Crosslinked alginic acid	Alginic acid NF, Satialgine
Natural super disintegrant	Soy polysaccharides, Emcosoy, Calcium silicate

2.6.5 Lubricants

Lubricants act by reducing friction by interposing an intermediate layer between the tablet constituents and the die wall during compression and ejection which would help tablet to easily eject from the die cavity and would prevent sticking of tablet to die cavity. It helps tablet to prevent from lamination, sticking and chipping. An ideal lubricant should reduce friction at small quantity.

Classification of lubricants

Lubricants are classified according to their water solubility (Hydrophilic, hydrophobic) and physical characteristics (Solid, fluid).

A Classification according to solubility

(a) *Hydrophilic lubricants*: Water soluble lubricants are used when a tablet is completely soluble or when unique disintegration and dissolution characteristics are required.

(b) *Hydrophobic lubricants*: Water insoluble lubricants are most effective and used at reduced concentration than water soluble lubricants. Since these lubricants function by coating.

B Classification according to physical characteristics

(a) *Solid lubricants*: Solid lubricants acts by boundary mechanism and are more effective and more frequently used. Example, Magnesium stearate.

(b) *Fluid lubrication*: Fluid lubricants acts by separating moving surfaces completely with a layer of lubricant and either added to the mix or applied directly to the die-wall. Disadvantage is that the oily lubricants may give a mottled tablet appearance due to uneven distribution. These are typically mineral oils or vegetable oils.

Various types of Lubricants along with their concentration are shown in Table 2.7.

TABLE 2.7

Types of lubricants

Insoluble lubricants	Concentration (%W/W)
Magnesium stearate	Up to 1%
Talc	1 to 5%
Stearic acid	1 to 5%
High melting waxes	3 to 5%
Maize starch	5 to 10%
Colloidal Silicon dioxide or aerosol	0.25 to 3%
Boric acid	1
Sodium oleate	5
Sodium benzoate	5
Polyethyene Glycol 4000	1 to 4
Polyethylene Glycol 6000	1 to 4
Sodium Lauryl Sulfate (SLS)	1 – 5

2.6.6 Anti Adherents

Anti adherent reduces adhesion of powder to punch faces and thus helps in preventing sticking. They are mostly used in combination with other lubricants to improve overall performance during compaction. Examples are talc, magnesium stearate and corn starch.

Types of anti adherents and their concentration range are shown in Table 2.8.

TABLE 2.8

Types of anti adherents

Anti adherent	Range (%W/W)
Talc	1 – 5
Cornstarch	3 – 10
Colloidal silica	0.1 – 0.5
DL-Leucine	3 – 10
Sodium lauryl sulfate	<1
Stearates	<1

2.6.7   Glidants

Glidants are added to the formulation to improve the flow properties of the powder or granules. It act correcting the surface irregularity, decreasing the surface charges and reducing the overall interparticulate friction of the system.

Examples of Glidants include magnesium stearate, talc, colloidal silica (Syloid), fumed silicon dioxide, hydrated sodium silioaluminate.

2.6.8   Antioxidants

Antioxidants are added in tablet formulation to protect drug from undergoing oxidation. Most commonly used antioxidants include ascorbic acid and their esters, alpha-tocopherol, ethylene diamine tetra acetic acid, sodium metabisulfite, sodium bisulfite, Butylated Hydroxy Toluene (BHT), Butylated Hydroxy Anisole (BHA), citric acid, and tartaric acid.

2.6.9 Preservatives

Preservatives may be a part of tablet formulation in order to prevent the growth of microorganisms in tablet formulation. Parabens like methyl, propyl, benzyl and butyl p-hydroxy benzoate are used as preservatives.

2.6.10 Sweeteners

Sweeteners are added primarily to chewable tablets. Sucrose is the most commonly used sweetener traditionally.

Saccharin is 500 times sweeter than sucrose. Its major disadvantages are that it has a bitter after taste and is carcinogenic.

Cyclamate is carcinogenic in nature.

Aspartame is about 200 times sweeter than sucrose. The primary disadvantage is that it is unstable in presence of moisture. When aspartame is used with hygroscopic components, it will be necessary to determine its stability under conditions in which the product can absorb atmospheric moisture

2.6.11 Colourants

Colourants are incorporated into tablets to enhance the aesthetic appearance of the product to have better patient acceptance. It also helps for the purpose of identification and to create brand image. Most widely used colorants are dyes and lakes which are FD & C and D & C approved as shown in Table 2.9.

TABLE 2.9

Types of FD & C Colour

FD & C Colour	Common name
Red 3	Erythrosine
Red 40	Allura red AC
Yellow 5	Tartrazine
Yellow 6	Sunset Yellow
Blue 1	Brilliant Blue
Blue 2	Indigotine
Green 3	Fast Green

2.6.12   Flavours

Flavours are commonly used to improve the taste of chewable tablets as well as mouth dissolved tablets. Flavours are incorporated either as solids (spray dried flavours), oils or aqueous (water soluble) flavours.

2.6.13   Co-processed Excipients

Co-processing means combining two or more materials by a suitable process to enhance tableting properties such as tablet strength, flow property and compressibility. Types of co-processed excipients are given in Table 2.10.

Example: Silified MCC is a blend of microcrystalline cellulose and colloidal silicon dioxide.

TABLE 2.10

Types of co-processed excipients

Trade name	Description
Cal-Tab®	Calcium sulfate 93% and vegetable gum 7%
Ludipress®	93% α-lactose monohydrate, 3.5% polyvinylpyrrolidone, and 3.5% crospovidone.
Microcellac®	75% lactose and 25% MCC (Micro Crystalline Cellulose)
Nu-Tab®	Sucrose 95-97%, invert sugar 3-4% and magnesium stearate 0.5%
Di-Pac®	Sucrose 97% and modified dextrins 3%
Sugartab®	Sucrose 90-93% and invert sugar 7-10%.
Emdex®	Dextrose 93-99% and maltose 1-7%

2.7   Tablet Compression

The compression is done either by single punch machine (stamping press) or by multi station machine (rotary press).

2.7.1   Components and Functioning of Rotary Tablet Compression Machine

The rotary compression machine consists of following components as given in Figure 2.3.

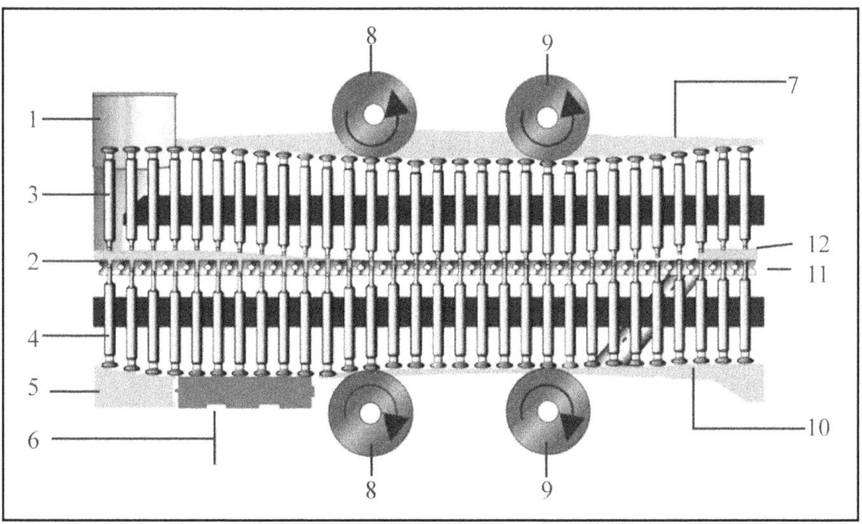

FIGURE 2.3 Component of rotary tablet compression machine.

1. **_Hopper_:** To hold and feed the granules.

2. **_Feed shoe_:** Provides feeding mechanism for the movement of granules from hopper to dies

3. **_Upper punches_:** For compression

4. **_Lower punches_:** For compression

5. **_Lower cam track_:** For guiding the movements of lower punches

6. **_Turrets_:** To hold the upper and lower punch

7. **_Upper cam track_:** For guiding the movements of upper punches

8. **_Pre-compression roller_:** This provides an initial compression force to granule to avoid air entrapment if any

9. **_Main-compression roller_:** This helps to apply compression force to formulate tablet

10. **_Ejection cam_:** This helps in ejection of tablet properly.

11. **_Die_:** To hold the powder/granules for compression.

12. **_Take-off blade_:** To remove tablet safely and intact.

A tablet machine output depends on

- Number of tooling set
- Number of compression cycle
- Rotational speed

The tablet press is a high-speed mechanical device. A tablet is made by pressing the granules or powder inside a die which is disc shaped with a hole cut through its centre. The powder is compressed in the centre of the die by upper and lower punches that fit into the top and bottom of the die. The punches and dies are fixed to a turret that spins round. As it spins, the punches are driven together by upper cam and lower cam. The punch head sits on the upper cam edge. The bottom of the lower punch sits on the lower cam edge.

Common process occurring during compression includes:

1. Filling
2. Compression and
3. Ejection

The basic stages of compression are shown in Figure 2.4.

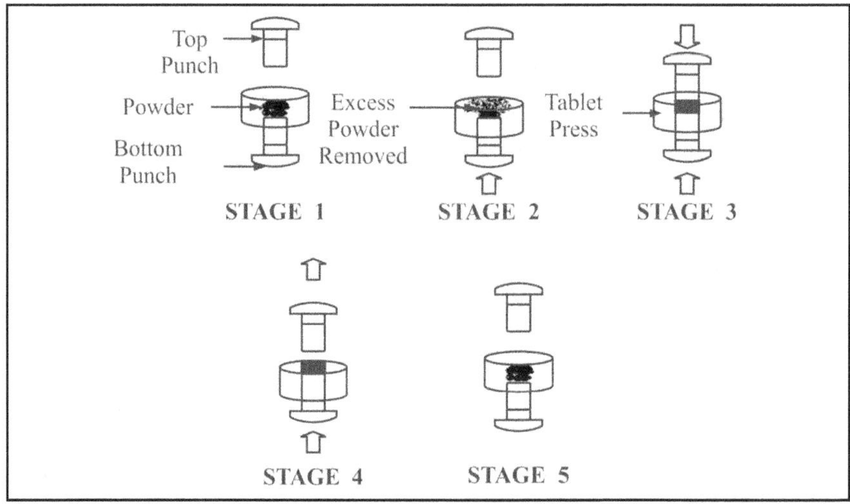

FIGURE 2.4 Stages of compression.

***Filling stage* 1:** Top punch is withdrawn from the die by the upper cam. Bottom punch is low in the die so powder falls in through the hole and fills the die.

***Weight and adjustment stage* 2:** Bottom punch moves up to adjust the powder weight; it raises and expels the excess powder.

***Compression stage* 3:** Top punch is driven into the die by upper cam. Bottom punch is raised by lower cam. Both punch heads pass between heavy rollers to compress the powder.

***Ejection stage* 4:** The upper cam withdraws top punch. Lower punch is pushed up and expels the tablet. Tablet is removed from the die surface by surface plate.

***Repeat stage* 5:** The entire process (stage 1-4) is repeated.

2.8   Evaluation of Tablets

The quantitative evaluation of a tablet's chemical, physical and bioavailability properties are important in the design of tablets and to monitor product quality.

Official Quality control tests for tablets (Compendia tests)

1. Uniformity of content of active ingredient (weight & content uniformity).
2. Disintegration test.
3. Dissolution test.
4. Friability test.

Non-Compendia tests

There are many tests that are frequently applied on tablets for which there are non-pharmacopoeial requirements but will form a part of manufacture's own product specifications like.

1. Tablet size / thickness/colour/odour/taste.
2. Tablet hardness.

2.8.1 General Appearance

The general appearance of tablets, its visual identity and elegance is essential for consumer acceptance, to control lot-to-lot uniformity, general tablet-to-tablet uniformity and for monitoring the production process. The control of general appearance involves measurement of attributes such as a tablet's size, shape, colour, presence or absence of odour, taste, surface textures, physical flaws and consistency.

2.8.2 Size and Shape

The shape and dimensions of compressed tablets are dimensionally monitored and controlled. At a constant compressive load, tablets thickness varies with changes in die fill, particle size distribution, packing of the powder mix being compressed, tablet weight, while with a constant die fill, thickness varies with variation in compressive load.

2.8.3 Thickness

The thickness of individual tablets may be measured with a micrometer, which gives accurate measurements and provides information regarding the variation between tablets. Sliding caliper scale is used to measure crown thickness by placing 5-10 tablets in a holding tray. Tablet thickness should be controlled within a standard value to facilitate packaging.

2.8.4 Colour

Non uniformity of colour is generally referred to as mottling. Non uniformity of colour not only lacks aesthetic appeal but could be associated by the consumer with non uniformity of content and general poor product quality. The eye cannot differentiate small differences in colour nor can it precisely define colour efforts have been made to perform quantitative colour evaluations. Reflectance spectrophotometry, tristimulus colorimetric measurements and micro reflectance photometer have been used to measure colour uniformity and gloss on a tablet surface.

2.8.5 Odour

Presence and absence of odour can provide an indication of the quality of tablets as the presence of an odour in a batch of tablets could indicate a stability problem, such as the characteristic odour of acetic acid in degrading aspirin tablets. Hence it is important for consumer acceptance.

2.8.6 Taste

Taste is also important for consumer acceptance of certain tablets (*e.g.* chewable tablets) and many companies utilize taste panels to judge the preference of different flavors and flavor levels in the development of a product. Taste preference is however subjective and the control of taste in the production of chewable tablets is usually based on the presence or absence of a specified taste.

2.8.7 Weight Variation

The USP has provided limits for the average weight of uncoated compressed tablets are given in Table 2.11. Twenty tablets are weighed individually and the average weight is calculated. The individual tablet weights are then compared to the average weight. Not more than two of the tablets must differ from the average weight No tablet must differ by more than double the relevant percentage. Weight variation requirement as per the USP and BP are as given in Table 2.11.

TABLE 2.11

Weight variation requirements as per USP and BP

USP		BP	
Average weight of tablet	Max % difference allowed	Average weight of tablet	Max % difference allowed
130 mg or less	10	80 mg or less	10
>130 mg and <324 mg	7.5	> 80 - < 250 mg	7.5
324 mg or more	5	> 250 mg	5

2.8.8 Hardness or Crushing Strength

Tablets should have certain amount of strength and resistance to friability to withstand mechanical shock of handling and transportation.

Monsanto or Stokes hardness tester measures the force required to break the tablet when the force is applied diametrally generated by a coil spring. The Strong-Cobb, Pfizer and Schleuniger apparatus measures the diametrically applied force required to break the tablet. The force required to break the tablet is measured in kilograms and a crushing strength of 4 Kg is usually considered to be the minimum for satisfactory tablets. If the tablet is too hard, it may not disintegrate in the required period of time to meet the dissolution specifications; if it is too soft, it may not be able to withstand the handling during subsequent processing such as coating or packaging and shipping operations. The hardness parameters for different types of tablets are given in Table 2.12.

Three measurable hardness parameters that will give indication to the strength and compactability are:

Bonding index: Higher the bonding index stronger is the tablet

Strain index: Higher the strain index weaker is the tablet

Brittleness Index: Higher brittleness index friability will be more

TABLE 2.12

Hardness parameter

Type of tablets	Hardness (kg/cm^2)
Oral conventional tablets	4-6
Hypodermic dispersible and chewable tablets	3-4
Sustained release tablets	8-20

2.8.9 Friability

The friability test is related with the tablet hardness and is determined to evaluate the ability of the tablet to withstand abrasion in packaging, handling and shipping. It is usually measured by the use of the Roche friabilator. 10 Tablets are weighed and placed in the plastic chamber which revolves at 50-100 rpm, where they are exposed to rolling and repeated shocks as they fall 6 inches in each turn within the apparatus. The tablets are reweighed and the weight compared with the initial weight. The loss due to abrasion is a measure of the tablet friability. The value is expressed as a percentage. A maximum weight loss of not more than 1% of the weight of the tablets is considered to be acceptable

2.8.10   Content Uniformity Test

To evaluate the tablet potential for efficacy, amount of drug in a tablet needs to be monitor from batch to batch. The content uniformity test is used to ensure that every tablet contains the amount of drug substance intended with little variation among tablets within a batch. USP defines content uniformity test for tablets containing 50 mg or less of drug substance in case of uncoated tablets and for all sugar coated tablets regardless of the drug content.

For content uniformity test, a representative sample of 30 tablets is selected randomly and 10 are assayed individually. (According to the method described in the individual monograph) The requirements for content uniformity are met if the amount of the active ingredient in each tablet lies within the range of 85-115% of the label claim and tenth tablet may not contain less than 75% and more than 125% of the label claim. If it does not meet the requirements, further 20 tablets are assayed individually and none of them should fall out of 85-115%.

2.8.11   Disintegration

The disintegration test is a measure of the time required under a given set of conditions for a group of tablets to disintegrate into particles which will pass through a 10 mesh screen. Generally, the test is useful as a quality assurance tool for conventional dosage forms. The test is carried out using the disintegration test apparatus which consists of a basket rack holding 6 plastic tubes, open at the top and bottom, the bottom of the tube is covered by a 10-mesh screen. The basket is immersed in a bath of suitable liquid held at 37°C, preferably in a 1L beaker. If 1 or 2 tablets fail to disintegrate, the test is repeated for 12 additional tablets; not less than 16 of the total of 18 tablets tested should disintegrate. For most uncoated tablets, the BP requires that the tablets disintegrate in 15 minutes while for coated tablets, up to 2 hours may be required.

2.8.12   Dissolution

Dissolution is the process by which a solid solute enters a solution. Dissolution is considered one of the most important quality control tests performed on pharmaceutical dosage forms. The principle function of the dissolution test is optimization of therapeutic effectiveness during product development and stability assessment, routine assessment of production quality to ensure uniformity between production lots, assessment of 'bioequivalence and prediction of '*in-vivo*' availability.

The various pharmacopoeias contain specifications on the dissolution requirements of various drugs. A variety of designs of apparatus for dissolution testing have been proposed and tested, varying from simple beaker with stirrer to complex systems as given in Table 2.13.

TABLE 2.13

Types of dissolution apparatus

	Pharmacopoeia			
Type	**USP**	**BP**	**IP**	**EP**
I	Rotating Basket	Rotating Basket	Rotating Paddle	Rotating Basket
II	Rotating Paddle	Rotating Paddle	Rotating Basket	Rotating Paddle
III	Reciprocating cylinder	Flow through cell	Flow through cell	
IV	Flow through cell			
V	Paddle over disc			
VI	Rotating cylinder			
VII	Reciprocating Disc			

The choice of the apparatus to be used depends largely on the physicochemical properties of the dosage form.

Apparatus I (Basket Type)

The assembly consists of a covered vessel of glass or other inert transparent material; a motor; a metallic drive shaft; and a cylindrical basket. The vessel is partially immersed in a suitable water bath of any convenient size or placed in a heating jacket. The water bath or heating jacket permits holding the temperature inside the vessel at $37 + 0.5^\circ$ during the test and keeping the bath fluid in constant, smooth motion.

The vessel is cylindrical, with a hemispherical bottom and with one of the following dimensions and capacities: for a nominal capacity of 1 L, the height is 160 mm to 210 mm and its inside diameter is 98 mm to 106 mm; for a nominal capacity of 2 L, the height is 280 mm to 300 mm and its inside diameter is 98 mm to 106 mm; and for a nominal capacity of 4 L, the height is 280 mm to 300 mm and its inside diameter is 145 mm to 155 mm. Its sides are flanged at the top. The shaft is positioned so that its axis is not more than 2 mm at any point from the vertical axis of the vessel and rotates smoothly and without significant wobble. A speed-regulating device is used that allows the shaft rotation speed to be selected and maintained at the rate specified in the individual monograph, and basket components of the stirring element are fabricated of stainless steel. The distance between the inside bottom of the vessel and the basket is maintained at $25 + 2$ mm during the test

Apparatus II (Paddle Type)

It is similar to the assembly from Apparatus 1, except that a paddle formed from a blade and a shaft is used as the stirring element. The paddle blade and shaft may be coated with a suitable inert coating. The dosage unit is allowed to sink to the bottom of the vessel before rotation of the blade is started. A small, loose piece of nonreactive material such as a helix wire, not more than a few turns, may be attached to dosage units that would otherwise float.

Unless otherwise specified in the individual monograph, the requirements are met if the quantities of active ingredient dissolved from the units tested confirm to the accompanying acceptance values. Continue testing through the three stages unless the results confirm at either S1 or S2 as depicted in Table 2.14. The quantity Q, is the amount of dissolved active ingredient specified in the individual monograph, expressed as a percentage of the labeled content; the 5%, 15%, and 25% values in the acceptance table are percentages of the labeled content so that these values and Q are in the same terms.

TABLE 2.14

Dissolution acceptance table

Stage	Number Tested	Acceptance Criteria
S1	6	Each unit is not less than Q + 5%.
S2	6	Average of 12 units (S1 + S2) is equal to or greater than Q, and no unit is less than Q − 15%.
S3	12	Average of 24 units (S1 + S2 + S3) is equal to or greater than Q, not more than 2 units are less than Q − 15%, and no unit is less than Q − 25%.

2.9 Tablet Processing Problems, Causes and their Solutions

The main source of the problem in tablet making is the formulations, the compression equipment or combination of both. The probable causes and remedies of tablet problems are shown in Table 2.15

TABLE 2.15

Problems, their causes and remedies of tablet defects

Problems	Definition	Causes	Remedies
Capping and Lamination	Partial or complete separation of the top or bottom parts of the tablet from the main body of the tablet.	High pressure of the punch - Deep concave punches - Air entrapment between the granules - Improper setup of the upper and lower punches - Too much dry granules - Addition of the hygroscopic substance	Alter the distance between the punches - Slowing the compression speed - Use of flat or less concave punches

*Table 2.15 **contd...***

Problems	Definition	Causes	Remedies
Lamination	The separation of the tablet into the two or more distinct layers.	- High speed of the compression - High temperature of the die - Over drying of the granules - Insufficient amount of the binding agent	- Reduce the speed of the compression machine - Change the punch set - Addition of the proper binder
Picking	Term used to describe the surface material from the tablet that is sticking to and being removed from the tablet's surface by a punch.	Due to the letters on the punch surface like A, B, M, R etc.	Proper design and larger size of letters - Larger size of the tablet - Use of colloidal silica as a polishing agent to the punch
Sticking	used to describe the material getting off from the tablet surface and adheres to the surface of the die.	- Low melting point of the substances - Insufficient and uneven lubrication - Under dried granules - Unpolished and rough surface of the punches	- Use of colloidal silica - Addition of high melting point substances - Use of air cooling - Addition of lubricants - Proper drying of granules - Use of new die-punch set
Mottling	Unequal distribution of the colour on a tablet with light and dark areas instead of the uniform distribution.	- Migration of the colour during drying - Due to colour difference between drugs and additives - Improper mixing of the colour	- Drying of granules at low temperature - Change of the solvent system - Use of the dye which mask the colour of the tablet ingredients

Table 2.15 *contd...*

Problems	Definition	Causes	Remedies
Weight Variation	difference in the weight of the tablets of the same batch.	- Poor granules flow - Under dried granules - Large portion of fines in the final granules - Different density distribution - Uneven distance between two punches and die - Pressure of the punch sets	- Slow compression speed - Use of proper glidants - Use of new sets of punches and die - Use of vibrator at the bottom part of the hopper
Double Impression:	During the free movement of the lower punch, the punch rotates in circular motion during compressing the tablet and ejecting it from the die. So, the tablet receives the imprint of the punch on its bottom surface. Similar problems can be encountered with engraved upper punches.	- Sticking of granules - Tooling set is improper	- Use of new punch and die set - Punches should be coated with cromium - Proper lubrication of the press parts

2.10 Recent Advancement of Tablet Technology

The recent advancement in tablet technology reduces the personnel input, material handling, processing steps of each unit operation thus ensuring enhance product quality and process reliability.

Advancement in Raw Materials

Recent advancements in material science such as, directly compressible vehicle, co processed and multiple use excipients helps to avoid multiple steps involved in the tablet manufacturing. This ready to use co-processed blends for direct compression reduces the processing time and improves quality of tablets. *E.g.* celllutab, Di pac, Indipress cellatose, Pharmatose DCL 40.

Advancement in Granulation Techniques

Various novel methods such as, Pneumatic Dry Granulation, freeze granulation Technology, Foamed Binder Technologies, Melt Granulation Technology, Steam Granulation and Thermal Adhesion Granulation

Process have replaced the conventional wet granulation method for automatic or semi-automatic production of granules.

Advancement in Equipment Technology

A major breakthrough in development of fully automatic instrumentation system to optimize each unit operation from mixing, granulation, slugging, compaction, and compression or most of the unit operation in one system. Recent technological advances have allowed the mixing, wetting, agglomeration and drying of tableting materials in a continuous process, all within a single instrument *E.g*: Rotary fluidized bed granulator/dryers, Mixer-processor & mixer-granulator with vacuum drying mechanism, Mixer-processor & mixer-granulator with fluidized bed drying mechanism.

Advancement in Compression Technology

The rotary tablet machines have been developed which are capable of producing one, two or three layered tablets, tablet in tablets, compression coated tablets etc. E.g. OSDrC® OptiDose™

Advancement as per Application

The recent advancements in tablet formulations include immediate release tablets such as orally dispersible mini tablets, mouth dissolving/fast dissolving tablets, conventional effervescent, melt in mouth tablets etc. modified release tablet formulations including layered tablets such as inlay tablets, tablet in tablet, bilayered tablet, medicated chewing gum, tablet tarts, pastilles, lollipop, tablet inserts, clinicaps, caplets and child ecstasy tablets.

Mouth Dissolving Tablets

Mouth-dissolving tablets also termed as: Fast disintegrating tablets melt-in-mouth, quick-dissolving, rapid dissolve, quick-disintegration, orally disintegrating, fast-melt, oro dispersible, and effervescent drug absorption system.

Inlay Tablets

 Inlay tablet is a type of layered tablet in which instead of the core tablet being completely surrounded by coating, the top surface is completely exposed.

Caplet

Caplets are the oblong-shaped tablet, alternative to the capsule that can be easily administered.

3 Tablet Coating

3.1 Tablet Coating

Drugs have their own characteristics, like many drugs are bitter in taste, obnoxious odour, light sensitive, or hygroscopic in nature. Tablet coating is the choice of option to solve such problems in conventional dosage form. The use of coating has as a process that originates from the time of the Egyptians. Sugar coating of pills was developed in the mid-1800s. Film coating is a new technology dating back to the 1950s. Tablet coating is the application of coating composition to moving bed of tablets with concurrent use of heated air to facilitate evaporation of solvent.

3.2 Reason for Coating

Coating as an additional step in the manufacturing process, increases the cost of the product; therefore, the reason to coat a tablet is based on the following objectives;

1. To protect the drug from the environment such as light and moisture with a view to improve its stability.
2. To mask the taste of a drug having a bitter taste or an unpleasant odour.
3. To facilitate handling in packaging lines.
4. To improve mechanical integrity by protecting from chipping and abrasion.
5. To incorporate another drug in the coating to avoid chemical incompatibility.
6. To modify the drug release profile of drug.
7. Easy identification of color coated tablet by manufacturer, patients.
8. To improve elegance.

Selection of coating process will depend on:

1. Type of tablets

2. Durability of core

3. Economy

4. Type of coating

3.3   Types of Tablet Coating Process

3.3.1 Sugar Coating

Sugar coating is a successive application of sucrose based solution to the tablet core. This is a traditional method used to mask the bitterness and flavour of particularly unpleasant tasting drugs. The other advantage of a sugar coating is protection from the environmental factors such as, light or moisture from affecting the drug's stability. It is a multistage process and involves following separate operations:

3.3.1.1 Sealing

To prevent moisture penetration and strengthen the tablet core seal coat is applied. The quantities of material applied as a sealant will depend primarily on the tablet size, batch size and porosity. Common materials used as a sealant include Shellac, Zein, cellulose acetate phthalate (CAP), polyvinyl acetate phthalate, Hyroxyl propyl cellulose, Hyroxy propyl methyl cellulose etc.

Shellac has disadvantage of impaired bioavailability by lengthening the disintegration and dissolution time due to change in the resin property during storage.

Improper sealing stage (over application) can lead to the disintegration problem.

3.3.1.2 Sub Coating

The sub coating is applied to round the edges and buildup the tablet size. This step consists of alternately applying a binder solution followed by a sub coating powder dusting, which also acts as the foundation for the smoothing and colour coats. This is a highly critical operation as weight buildup occurs here. Generally, two methods are used for sub coating, first the repetitive application of gum based solution followed by dusting with powder and then drying. This routine is repeated until the desired shape is achieved. The second is the application of a suspension of dry powder in gum/sucrose solution followed by drying. The typical formulas are as shown in Table 3.1.

TABLE 3.1

Binder solution, dusting powder and suspension formulation for sub coating

Binder solution		Dusting powder		Suspension sub coating	
Ingredients	%W/W	Ingredients	%W/W	Ingredients	%W/W
Gelatin	6	Calcium carbonate	40.0	Sucrose	40.0
Gum acacia	8	Titanium dioxide	5.0	Calcium carbonate	20.0
Sucrose	45	Talc, asbestos free	25.0	Talc, asbestos free	12.0
Distilled water	Up to 100	Sucrose	28.0	Gum acacia(powdered)	2.0
		Gum acacia	2.0	Titanium dioxide	1.0
				Distilled water	25.0

3.3.1.3 Grossing/Smoothing

The grossing/smoothing process is for smoothing and filing the imperfection in the surface caused during sub coating. Smoothing usually can be accomplished by the application of three coats as;

(i) Grossing syrup

(ii) Heavy syrup

(iii) Regular syrup

Smoothing usually can be carried out by the application of a simple syrup solution (approximately 60-70 % sugar solid). This syrup generally contains pigments, starch, gelatin, acacia or opacifier if required.

3.3.1.4 Colouring

This stage is often critical in the successful completion of a sugar coating process. To attain final smoothness, required size and the required color several coats of a thin syrup containing color are applied. In the final finishing step, a few clear coats of syrup may be applied.

Mainly soluble dyes and water insoluble pigments were used in the sugar coating process to achieve the desired color. But now-a-days the insoluble pigments such as aluminum lakes or iron oxides have replaced the soluble dyes as they are easier to use and permit fast colour.

3.3.1.5 Polishing

Sugar-coated tablets need to be polished to achieve a desired luster. Polishing is achieved by applying the mixture of waxes like beeswax, carnauba wax, candelilla wax or hard paraffin wax to tablets in polishing pan.

Problems involved in sugar coating:

1. Increase in weight of tablet if proper care is not exercised.
2. Over use of dusting powder in sub coating stage results in the formation of soft and crack coating.
3. Washing back due to over dosing of colored syrup as previous coating redissolves.
4. Colour migration.
5. Rough tablets produced during the process may give marbled appearance during polishing.

Disadvantages

1. Tedious and time consuming method requires several days.
2. Specialized, highly skilled technicians are required.
3. Increases size and weight of tablet (50-100).

3.3.2 Film Coating

Film coating is deposition of a thin film of polymer surrounding the tablet core. The process of formation of film involves three steps as shown in Figure 3.2

(a) Latex particles dispersed in aqueous phase

(b) Formation of thin film with water evaporation through film

(c) Formation of continuous film

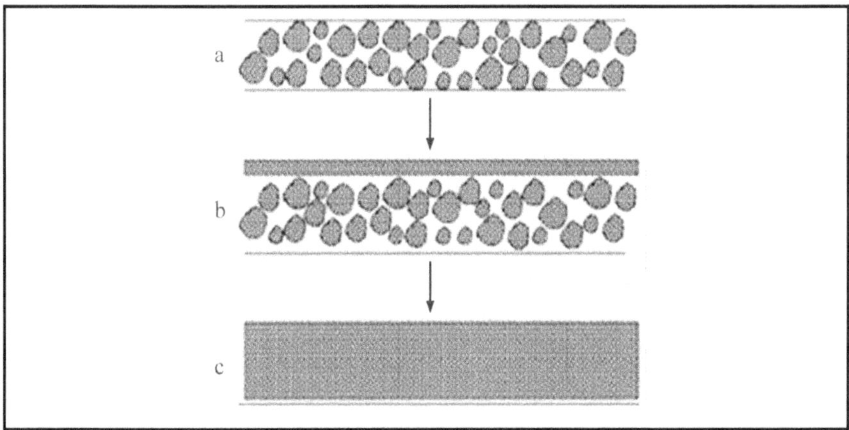

FIGURE 3.1 Process of formation of film.

3.3.2.1 Ideal Characters of Coating Material

- Essentially no odour or taste of its own.
- Solubility in the solvent of choice.
- Capacity to produce elegant product.
- Stability in presence of water, heat, moisture and air.
- No change in properties with aging.
- Compatibility with coating solution additives.
- Nontoxic and ease of application.
- Resistance to cracking.
- No bridging or filling of the debossed tablet surfaces by the film former.
- Ease of printing.

3.3.2.2 Materials used in Film Coating

1. Film formers
2. Solvents
3. Plasticizers
4. Colorants
5. Opaquant-Extenders
6. Miscellaneous coating solution components

I. Film Formers

Ideal requirements of film coating materials are:

- Solubility in solvent of choice
- Solubility requirement for the intended use e.g. free water-solubility, slow water-solubility or pH-dependent solubility
- Capacity to produce an elegant product
- Stable against heat, light, moisture, air
- No inherent color, taste or odor of its own
- High compatibility with other additives
- Nontoxic with no pharmacological activity
- High resistance to cracking
- should not give bridging or filling of the debossed tablet
- Compatible to printing procedure
- Film properties should not change on ageing

A. Non Enteric Polymers

(a) *Hydroxy Propyl Methyl Cellulose* **(HPMC):** The polymer is prepared by reacting alkali treated cellulose with methyl chloride to introduce methoxy group and then with propylene oxide to introduce propylene glycol ether groups. It is available in different viscosity grades. It is a polymer of choice for air suspension and pan spray coating systems.

It does not affect tablet disintegration and drug availability, it is cheap, flexible, chip resistance highly resistant to heat, light and moisture, it has no taste and odour, colour and other additives can be easily incorporated.

Solubility in gastrointestinal fluid, aqueous and organic solvents.

These have some disadvantages like, the polymer has tendency to bridge or fill the debossed tablet, surfaces. So mixture of HPMC and other polymers/ plasticizers are used.

(b) *Methyl Hydroxy Ethyl Cellulose*: This polymer is prepared by alkali treated cellulose with methyl chloride and then with ethylene oxide. It is available in wide variety of viscosity grades. It is not frequently used as HPMC because it is soluble in relatively fewer organic solvents.

(c) ***Ethyl Cellulose (EC):*** It is prepared by reaction of ethyl chloride or sulfate with cellulose dissolved in sodium hydroxide. Depending on the degree of ethoxy substitution, different viscosity grades are available. It is completely insoluble in water and gastric fluids; hence it is used in combination with hydrophilic polymers like HPMC. Aqua coat is aqueous polymeric dispersion utilizing ethyl cellulose. These pseudolatex systems contain high solid content, low viscosity compositions that have coating properties quite different from regular ethyl cellulose solution. It offers various processing advantages over organic ethyl cellulose solution, including reduced coating processing time, avoidance of potential toxicity due to residual solvent, and reduced environmental concerns.

The advantages of this polymer are soluble in wide variety of organic solvents, non-toxic, colourless, odourless and tasteless. These are stable in environmental condition.

Sometimes ethyl cellulose polymers are not preferred because, it is completely insoluble in water and gastric fluids it cannot be used alone, hence it is used in combination with water-soluble additives like HPMC. Ethyl cellulose films are brittle and require film modifiers to obtain an acceptable film formulation

(d) ***Hydroxy Propyl Cellulose:*** It is prepared by reaction of alkali treated cellulose with propylene oxide at high temperature. It is soluble in water below 40 °C and above it is insoluble. It is also soluble in gastric fluids and many polar organic solvents. It is extremely tacky as it dries from solution system. This polymer gives very flexible film.

(e) ***Povidone:*** Povidone is a synthetic polymer consisting of linear 1-vinyl-2 pyrrolidinone group. Degree of polymerization decides molecular weight of material. It is available in four viscosity grades i.e., K-15, K-30, K-60 and K-90. Average molecular weight of these grades is 10000, 40000, 160000 and 360000 respectively. K-30 is widely used as tablet binder and in tablet coating. It has excellent solubility in wide variety of organic solvents, water, gastric and intestinal fluids. Povidone can be cross-linked with other materials to produce films with enteric properties. It is used to improve dispersion of colourants in coating solution.

(f) ***Sodium Carboxy Methyl Cellulose:*** It is prepared by treating soda cellulose with sodium salt of monochloracetic acid. It is available in medium, high and extra high viscosity grades. It is easily dispersed in water to form colloidal solutions but it is insoluble in most organic solvents and hence not a material of choice for coating solution based on organic solvents. It produces brittle film but adhere well to tablets. Partially dried films of sodium carboxy methyl cellulose are tacky, so coating compositions must be modified with additives.

(g) ***Polyethylene Glycols***: It is prepared by reaction of ethylene glycol with ethylene oxide in presence of sodium hydroxide at elevated temperature and pressure. Different grades are available depending on the viscosity. Lower molecular weights PEG (200-600) are liquid at room temperature and are used as plasticizers. High molecular weight Polyethylene Glycol (PEGs) (900-8000 series) are white, waxy solids at room temperature. Combination of PEG waxes with Cellulose Acetate Phthalate (CAP) gives films that are soluble in gastric fluids.

(h) ***Acrylate Polymers***: It is marketed under the trademarks of Eudragit. Eudragit E is cationic polymer freely soluble in gastric fluid up to pH 5 and expandable and permeable above pH 5. This material is available as:

- Organic solution (12.5% in isopropanol/acetone),
- Solid material
- 30% aqueous RL®dispersion.

Eudragit RL & RS are co-polymers synthesized from acrylic and methacylic esters with low content of quaternary ammonium groups. These are available only as organic solutions and solid materials. They produce films for delayed action (pH dependent).

B. Enteric Polymers

(a) *Reason for Enteric Coating*

- To protect acid labile drugs e.g. enzymes
- To prevent from gastric distress and nausea e.g. sodium salicylate
- To deliver drugs intended for local action in intestine
- To provide delayed release

(b) *Ideal Properties of Enteric Coating Material are*

- Resistance to gastric fluids
- Susceptible/permeable to intestinal fluid
- Compatibility with most coating solution components and the drug substrate
- Formation of continuous film
- Nontoxic, cheap and ease of application

Polymers used for enteric coating are as follow:

1. *Cellulose Acetate Phthalate* (*CAP*): CAP is widely used polymer in the industry. It has the disadvantage of dissolving above pH 6 only, delays absorption of drugs. It is hygroscopic and permeable to moisture in comparison with other enteric polymer, it is susceptible to hydrolytic removal of phthalic and acetic acid changing film properties. CAP films are brittle and usually used with other hydrophobic film forming materials

   Aquateric is reconstituted colloidal dispersion of latex particles, composed of solid or semisolid polymer spheres of CAP ranging in size from 0.05 - 3 microns.

2. *Acrylate Polymers*: Eudragit L and Eudragit S are two forms of commercially available enteric acrylic resins. Both of them produce films resistant to gastric fluid. Eudragit L and S are soluble in intestinal fluid at pH 6 and 7 respectively. Eudragit L is available as an organic solution (Isopropanol), solid or aqueous dispersion. Eudragit S is available only as an organic solution (Isopropanol) and solid.

3. *Hydroxy Propyl Methyl Cellulose Phthalate*: It is prepared by esterification of HPMC with phthalic anhydride. HPMCP 50, 55 & 55-s (also called HP-50, HP-55 & HP-55-s) is widely used. HP-55 is recommended for general enteric preparation while HP-50 & HP-55-s for special cases. These polymers dissolve at a pH 5-5.5.

4. *Polyvinyl Acetate Phthalate*: It is prepared by the esterification of partially hydrolyzed polyvinyl acetate with phthalic anhydride. It is similar to HP-55 in stability and pH dependent solubility.

II. Solvents

Solvents are used to dissolve or disperse the polymers and other additives and convey them to substrate surface.

Ideal requirements are:

- Should be either dissolved or dispersed polymer system
- Should easily disperse other additives
- Small concentration of polymers (2-10%) should not create processing problems in an extremely viscous solution system
- Should be colourless, tasteless, odourless, inexpensive, inert, nontoxic and nonflammable
- Rapid drying rate
- No environmental pollution.

Mostly solvents are used either alone or in combination with water, ethanol, methanol, isopropanol, chloroform, acetone, methylene chloride, etc. Water is more used because no environmental and economic considerations are involved. For drugs that readily hydrolyze in presence of water, non-aqueous solvents are preferable.

III. Plasticizers

Plasticizers are simply relatively low molecular weight materials which are added to alter the physical properties of the polymer to render it more useful in performing its function as a film-coating material. As solvent is removed, most polymeric materials tend to pack together in three dimensional honey comb arrangement. Plasticizers are used to modify quality of film. Concentration of plasticizer is expressed in relation to the polymer being plasticized. Commonly used plasticizers are castor oil, propylene glycol, glycerin, lower molecular weight poly ethylene glycol, surfactants, etc. For aqueous coating PEG and PG are more used while castor oil and spans are primarily used for organic-solvent based coating solution. The plasticizer and the film former must be at least partially soluble or miscible with each other.

IV. Colourants

Colourants can be used in solution form or in suspension form. They are used to provide distinctive color and elegance to the product. To achieve proper distribution of suspended colorants in the coating solution the use of the powdered colorants is required (<10 microns). Most common colorants in use are certified FD & C or D & C colourants. These are synthetic dyes or lakes. Lakes are choice for sugar or film coating as they give reproducible results. Concentration of colorants in the coating solutions depends on the color shade desired, the type of dye, and the concentration of opaquant-extenders. If very light shade is desired, concentration of less than 0.01 % may be adequate on the other hand, if a dark color is desired a concentration of more than 2.0 % may be required. The inorganic materials (*e.g.* iron oxide) and the natural coloring materials (*e.g.* anthrocyanins, carotenoids, etc.) are also used to prepare coating solution

V. Opaquant-Extenders

These are very fine inorganic powder used to provide more pastel colours and increase film coverage. These inorganic materials provide white coat or mask colour of the tablet core. Colourants are very expensive and higher concentration is required but these inorganic materials are cheap. In presence of these inorganic materials, amount of colourants required decreases. Most commonly used materials are titanium dioxide, silicate (talc & aluminum silicates), carbonates (magnesium carbonates), oxides (magnesium oxide) & hydroxides (aluminum hydroxides).

VI. Miscellaneous Coating Solution Component

(a) *Flavours and sweeteners* are used to mask unpleasant odours or to develop the desired taste. For example, aspartame, various fruit spirits (organic solvent), water soluble pineapple flavour (aqueous solvent) etc.

(b) *Surfactants* are used to solubilize immiscible or insoluble ingredients in the coating. *For example*: Spans, Tweens etc.

(c) *Antioxidants* are incorporated to stabilize a dye system to oxidation and colour change. *For example*: Oximes, Phenols etc.

(d) *Antimicrobials* are added to put off microbial growth in the coating composition. Some aqueous cellulosic coating solutions are mainly prone to microbial growth, and long-lasting storage of the coating composition should be avoided. *For example*: alkyl isothiazloinone, carbamates, benzothiazoles etc.

3.4   Coating Process

Film-coating of tablets is a multivariate process, with many different factors, such as coating equipment, coating liquid, and process parameters which affect the pharmaceutical quality of the final product. Film coating of tablets are carried out by a pan pour method, pan spray process and fluidized method.

3.4.1 Pan-Pour Method

Tablet coated by pan pour methods involves alternate solution application, mixing and drying.

Disadvantages

1. Slow and relies on the skill and techniques of operator.
2. Requires additional drying steps.
3. Aqueous based film coatings are not suitable.

3.4.2 Pan-Spray Method

Spraying leads to automated control of liquid application.

3.4.3 Fluidized Bed Process

Fluidized bed system has been used for rapid coating of tablets, granules and beads held in suspension by a column of air. Adequate fluidization and drying depends on the volume and rate of processed air.

3.5 Components of Tablet Coating System

There are 3 primary components of tablet coating:

1. Tablet properties.
2. Coating process.
   - Coating equipment
   - Parameters of the coating process
   - Facility and ancillary equipment
   - Automation in coating process.
3. Coating composition

3.5.1 Tablet Properties

1. Tablet must be resistant to abrasion and chips.
2. The ideal shape of the tablet for coating is sphere.
3. The hardness of the tablet should not be less than 5 kg/cm^2.
4. The tablet must have good friability.
5. Tablets must have good flow.

3.5.2 Coating Process

The basic principle of tablet coating is simple. Tablet coating is an application of coating composition to a moving bed of tablets with the concurrent use of heated air to facilitate evaporation of the solvent. The distribution of coating is accomplished by the movement of the tablets either perpendicular (coating pan) or vertical (air suspension).

3.5.2.1 Coating Equipments

- It includes Coating pan, Spraying system, Air Handling System. Dust collector and Controls as Shown in Figure 3.2.

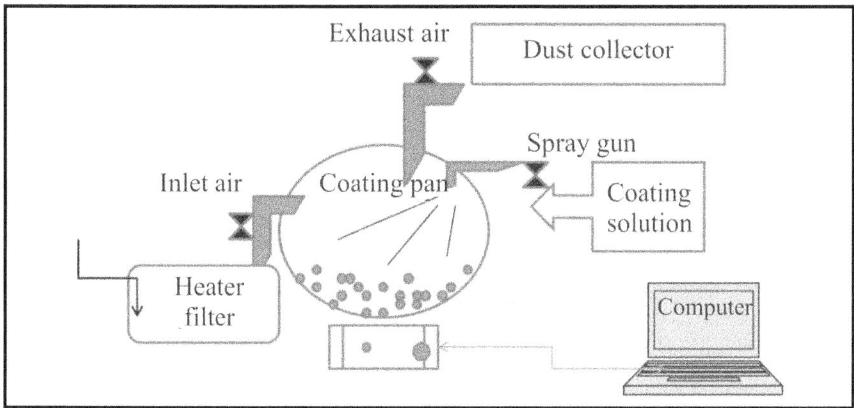

FIGURE 3.2 Coating equipments.

3.5.2.1.1 Coating Pan

The coating pan is actually a perforated drum that rotates within a cabinet. The cabinet enables you to control airflow, air temperature, air pressure, and the coating application.

There are three types of equipment generally available:

1. ***Standard coating pan***
   - Pellegrin pan system
   - Immersion sword system
   - Immersion tube system
2. ***Perforated pan system***
   - Accela cota system
   - Hicoater system

- Glattcoater system
- Driacoated system

3. *Fluidized bed coater*

- High pressure airless systems
- Low pressure air atomized systems

The schematic diagram of process of fluidized bed coating is depicted in Fig. 3.3.

1. ***Standard coating pan:*** It consists of a circular metal pan mounted angularly on the stand. The pan is 8 to 60 inches in diameter and is rotated on its horizontal axis by a motor. Hot air is directed into the pan and onto the tablet bed surface and is exhausted by means of the ducts positioned through the front of the pan. Coating solution is applied on to the tablets by hand pour or spraying the material onto the rotating tablet bed by using atomized systems (Figure 3.3). The drawback of standard coating pan is the poor drying efficiency which can be improved by pellegrini, immersion sword and immersion tube systems (Figure 3.3).

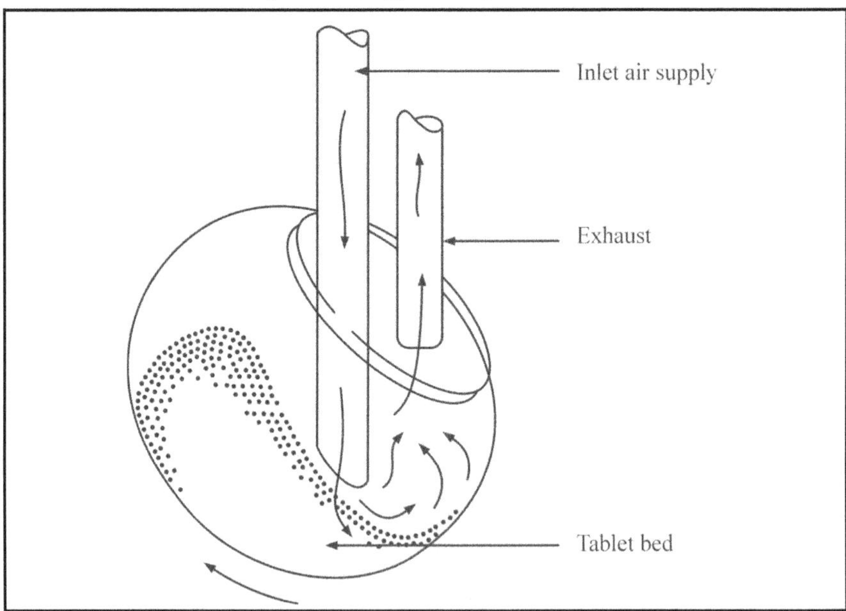

FIGURE 3.3 Standard coating pan.

- ***Pellegrin pan system*:** This system has a baffled pan and a diffuser that distributes the drying air uniformly over the tablet bed surface.

- ***Immersion sword system*:** In this system drying air is introduced through a perforated metal sword device that is immersed in the tablet bed.

- ***Immersion tube system*:** In this the tube is immersed into the tablet bed. The tube delivers the heated air and the spray nozzle is built in the tip of the tube. The drying air flows upward through the tablet bed and is exhausted by the duct. Coating solution is applied simultaneously with the heated air from the immersed tube during the operation.

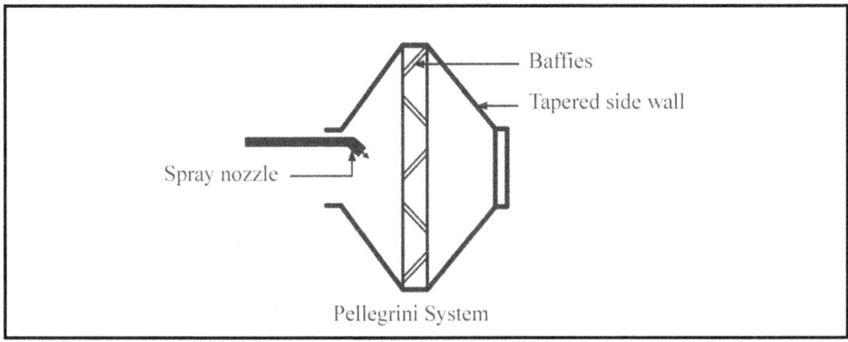

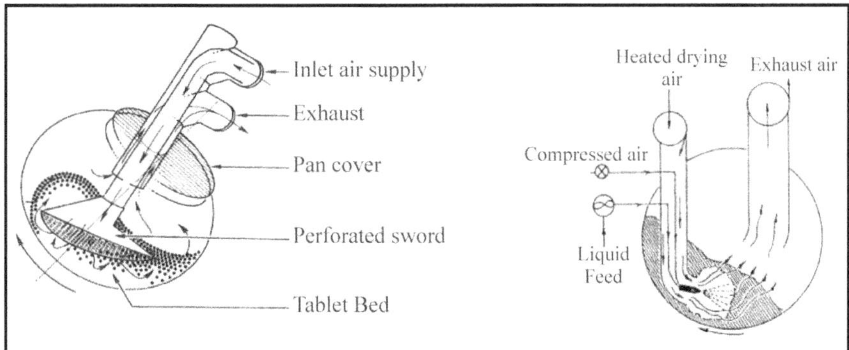

FIGURE 3.4 Standard coating pan system.

2. ***Perforated pan system*:** This consists of perforated or partially perforated drum that is rotated on its horizontal axis in an enclosed housing as shown in Figure 3.5. In all these four perforated pan systems the coating solution is applied to the surface of the rotating

bed of the tablets through spraying nozzles that are positioned inside the drum

- *Accela cota system and hicoater system***:** In these equipment the drying air is directed into the drum, is passed through the tablet bed and is exhausted through perforations in the drum

- *Glatt coater system***:**   It is the latest perforated pan coater. The drying air can be directed from the inside drum through the tablet bed and out an exhaust duct. Alternately, with an optional split plenum drying air can be directed in the reverse manner through the drum perforation for partial fluidization of tablet bed.

- *Dria coater system***:** In this the drying air is introduced through the hollow ribs located on the inside periphery of the drum. As the coating pan rotates the rib dip into the tablet bed and drying air passes through the tablet bed and is fluidized exhaust is from the back of the pan.

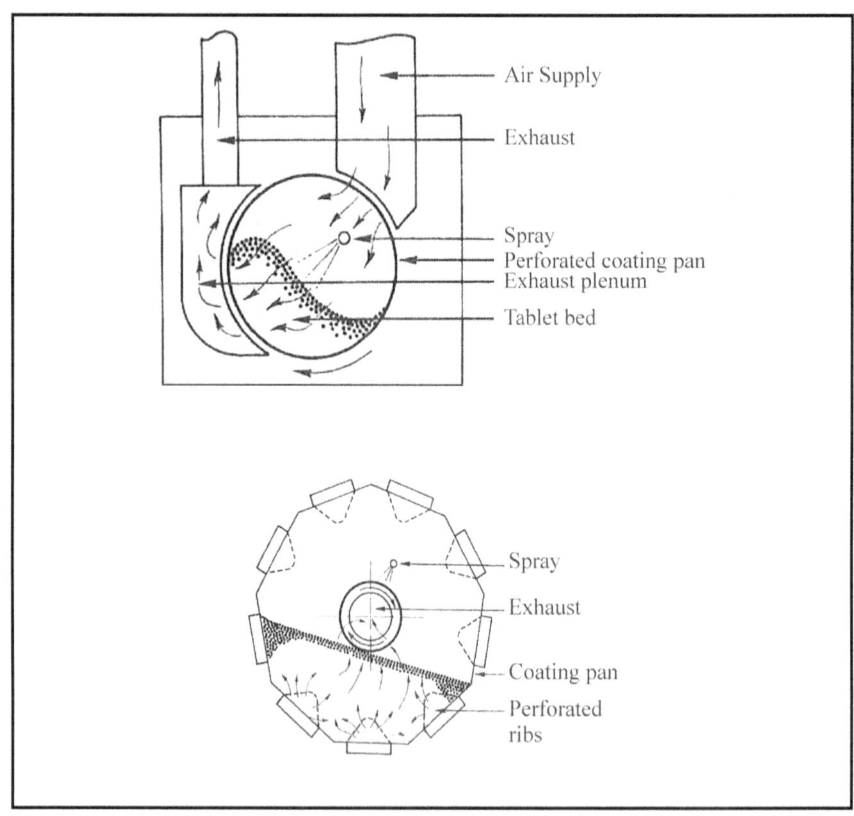

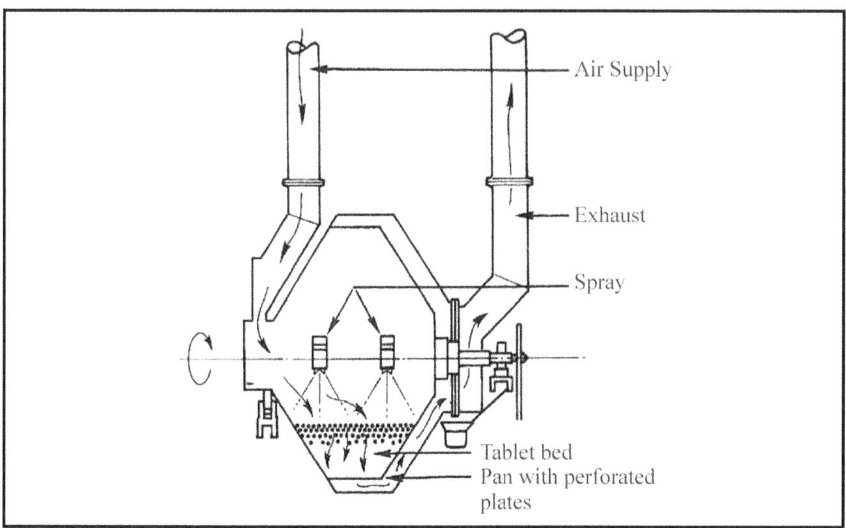

FIGURE 3.5 Types of perforated coating pan.

3. ***Fluidized bed coater*:** Fluidization of tablet bed is achieved in a columnar chamber by the upward flow of drying air. The airflow is controlled so that more air enters the center of the column, causing the tablets to buoyant in the centre. They then fall towards the chamber wall and move downward to re-enter the airstream at the bottom column is used to direct the tablet movement within the main column. Coating solutions are continuously applied from the spray nozzles located at the bottom of the chamber and sprayed on to the top of the cascading tablet bed by nozzles located in the upper region of the chamber (Figure 3.6).

The two types of systems used to apply a finely divided spray coating solutions or suspensions onto the tablets.

- ***High pressure airless systems:*** In this air less spray liquid is pumped at high pressure (250 to 3000 pounds per square inch gauge) through a small orifice (0.009 inch to 0.02 inch in diameter) in the fluid nozzle which results in a finely divided spray.

  The degree of the atomization and the spray rate are controlled by the fluid pressure, orifice size and viscosity of the liquid.

- ***Low pressure air atomized systems:*** In this the liquid is pumped through somewhat larger orifice (0.02 to 0.06 inch in diameter) at relatively low pressure (5 to 50 psig). Low pressure

(10 to 100 psig) air contacts the liquid stream at the tip of the atomizer and a finely divided spray is produced.

The degree of atomization is controlled by the fluid pressure, fluid cap orifice, viscosity of the fluid, air pressure and the air cap design.

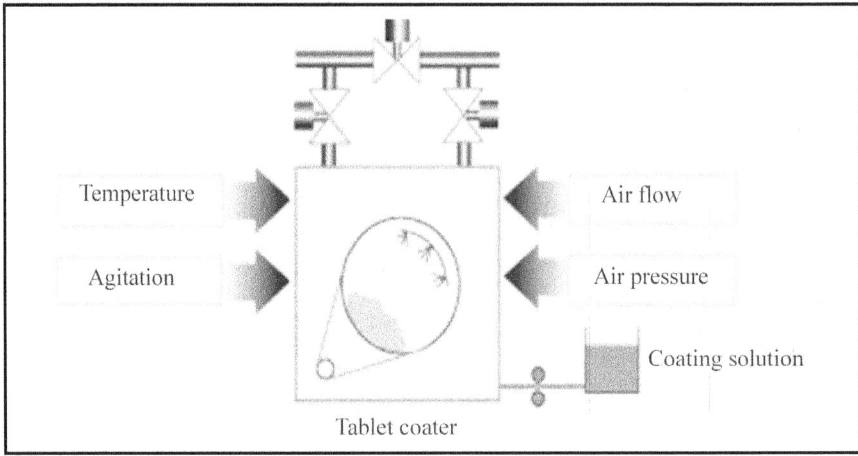

FIGURE 3.6 The schematic diagram of process of fluidized bed coating.

3.5.2.1.2　Spraying System

The spraying system consists of several spray guns mounted on a manifold, a solution pump, a supply tank and mixer, and an air supply.

The types of spray pattern include:

(a)　Top spray

(b)　Bottom spray

(c)　Tangential spray

The pump delivers the coating solution to the guns, where it combines with atomizing air to create a fine mist that is directed at the bed of tablets in the coating pan. The air handling unit heats and filters the air used to dry the coating on the tablets. The dust collector extracts air from the coating pan and keeps a slightly negative pressure within the cabinet. The controls enable you to control operation of all the components.

3.5.2.1.3　Air Handling System

Air handling unit includes, heaters, filters, Inlet air and exhaust air duct with valve, to provide the precise flow and validated quality of conditioned, drying air to maintain the most desirable coating conditions. These systems are used to meet the desired values of inlet air temperature and Humidity.

3.5.2.1.4   Dust Collectors

Hazardous contaminants generated by coating processes dictate the use of dust collectors to protect environments and personnel. The dust collector enhances performance, safety and ease of maintenance while protecting the workplace and environment.

3.5.2.1.5   Control Systems

It is the 'Brain' of the coating system. Advanced coating systems uses computer software to monitor a number of parameters, such as the temperature of the inlet and outlet air, humidity, rotation speed, spray rate, spray pattern, droplet size and thus ensures batch to batch consistency and quality.

3.5.2.2   Parameters of Coating Process

The variables to be controlled in pan spray film coating process are:

3.5.2.2.1   Quality of Tablets

The initial quality of tablets plays an important role for uniform coating. The tablets must be consistent in porosity, surface, moisture content and hardness. They must also be free of dust. Furthermore, they must not break apart during the preheat cycle at the start of the coating process or during the first few minutes of exposure to the atomized solution. If the surface of the tablet is too soft, the impingement of the solution can erode the tablet. Too hard a surface will not allow the solution to impinge and adhere, and the coating will peel away. The total surface area for unit weight decreases significantly from smaller to larger tablets. Application of a film with the same thickness requires less coating composition. In the coating process only a portion of the total surface is coated. Continuous partial coating and recycling eventually results in fully coated tablets.

3.5.2.2.2   Coating Liquid

The coating contains ingredients that are to be applied on the tablet surface and solvents, which act as carrier for the ingredients. Coating liquid, may affect the final quality of the tablets. Different film former has different chemical nature and different characteristic. Viscosity may affect the spreading of coating liquid across surface of substrate. Surface tension may affect in wetting of surface.

3.5.2.2.3 Pan Variables

1. Pan design/baffling
2. Speed
3. Load

Pan shape, baffling rotational speed, and loading effect the mixing of the tablet mass. Uniform mixing is essential to deposit the same quantity and quality of film on each tablet. Tablet shape may affect mixing as many shapes require a specific baffling system to ensure uniform mixing. Baffles if not properly selected may be a source for chipping and breaking. The pan speed effects the time the tablets spent on the spraying zone and, subsequently, the homogeneous distribution of the coating solution on the surface of each tablet throughout the batch. Pan speed that are too slow may cause localized over wetting, which leads to sticking of the tablets. Pan speed that is too high results in rough coating on the tablets due to non-uniform deposition of coating solution and also cause the tablet to undergo unnecessary attrition and breakage.

3.5.2.2.4 Spray Variables

1. Spray Rate
2. Spray pattern
3. Degree of atomization
4. Nozzel to bed distance

1. ***Spray rate***: The spray rate is a significant parameter since it impacts the moisture content of the formed coating and, subsequently, the quality and uniformity of the film. A low coating liquid spray rate causes incomplete coalescence of polymer due to insufficient wetting, which could effect in brittle films. A high coating liquid spray rate may result in over wetting of the tablet surface and subsequent problems such as picking and sticking. If the spray rate is high and the tablet surface temperature is low, films are not formed during the spraying but the post drying phase, and rapid drying often produces cracks in the films.

2. ***Spray pattern***: Wide spray pattern leads to loss of material and hence lower efficiency. Narrow spray pattern leads to localized over wetting and non-uniform coating.

3. ***Degree of atomization***: Atomization is a process where liquid is finely subdivided into droplets.

Degree of atomization is affected by:

1. Orifice size
2. Nozzle configuration
3. Fluid pressure
4. Air pressure
5. Fluid viscosity

In general, increasing the spraying air pressure decreases the surface roughness of coated tablets and produces denser and thinner films. If spraying air pressure is excessive, the spray loss is great, the formed droplets are very fine and could spray-dry before reaching the tablet bed, resulting in inadequate droplet spreading and coalescence. If spraying air pressure is inadequate, the film thickness and thickness variation are greater possibly due to change in the film density and smaller spray loss. In addition, with low spraying air pressure big droplets could locally over wet the tablet surface and cause tablets to stick to each other. Atomization that is too fine causes droplets to dry before reaching the tablet bed resulting in "spray drying" which leads to roughness.

Process air variable

1. Temperature
2. Volume of air
3. Air flow rate
4. Quality
5. Capacity

The inlet air temperature affects the drying efficiency of the coating pan and the uniformity of coatings. High inlet air temperature increases the drying efficiency of the aqueous film coating process and a decrease in the water penetration into the tablet core which decreases the core tablet porosity, tensile strength and residual moisture content of coated tablets. Too much air temperature increases the premature drying of the spray during application and, subsequently, decreases the coating efficiency. Measuring the pan air temperature helps to manage the optimum conditions during the coating process and, consequently, enables predicting possible drying or over wetting problems which may result in poor appearance of the film or may have unfavorable effects on the moisture and heat sensitive tablet cores.

The quantity of water or solvent that can be removed during the coating process depends on the quantity of air flowing through the tablet bed, temperature of the air and quantity of water that the inlet air contains. The balance between supply and exhaust air flow should be such that all dust and solvent are contained within the coating system.

4. *Nozzle to bed distance*: In most cases, the spray nozzle to bed distance should be optimum (6 in. to 10 inch), although the ideal distance depends on the force of the atomization, air pressure and coating pan size.

   If the distance between the nozzle and bed is less than the optimum, the wet droplets get deposited on the tablet surface and can cause surface wetting, leading to sticking of tablets. If the distance if more than the optimum than it causes the droplet to dry completely before reaching the tablet surface leading to spray drying condition and as the droplet hits the tablet surface in the dry powder form and it will not be able to make a continuous film.

3.5.2.2.5   Coating Efficiency

It is generally defined as a measure of the determined actual coating applied and is expressed as a percentage of the theoretical amount of coating intended to be applied. Ideally, 90-95% of the applied film coating should be on the tablet surface. Coating efficiency for conventional sugar coating is much less and 60% would be acceptable.

3.5.2.3 Facility and Ancillary Equipment

The facility required for any coating operation should be designed as per the requirements of Current Good Manufacturing Practices (CGMPs). Sufficient space is needed for the coating equipment, coating solution preparation and storage. The safety parameters should be considered where use of explosive or toxic concentrations of organic solvents occurs and hence, electrical explosion proofing, specialized ventilation are required for the same. Exhaust air treatment may be done to recover solvent or to prevent entry in to atmosphere.

Other Equipments needed to support the coating operation are Tanks, filters, mixers, mills, portable pressure tanks or pumping systems.

3.5.2.4 Automation

It involves the development of a process in which all the important variables are pre-programmed. With the help of sensors and regulating devices, temperature, airflow, spray rate, pan speed and a feed back control of the process is maintained.

3.5.3 Coating Composition

Most of the coating composition is solvent, so rapid removal is necessary to prevent undesirable effects on integrity of the tablets. Thin, rapid drying coating composition which dries quickly on the tablet surface is preferable. It includes Polymers, Solvents, Plasticizers, Colourants and Opaquant Extenders as already discussed in 3.2.2.2.

3.6 Process Design Control

Coating Process Design and Control: Tablet coating takes place in a controlled atmosphere inside a conventional/perforated rotating drum. Angled baffles fitted into the drum and air flow inside the drum provides means of mixing the tablet bed. As a result, the tablets are lifted and turned from the sides into the centre of the drum, exposing each tablet surface to an even amount of deposited/sprayed coating. The liquid spray coating is then dried onto the tablets by heated air drawn through the tablet bed from an inlet fan. The air flow is regulated for temperature and volume to provide controlled drying and extracting rates, and at the same time, maintaining the drum pressure slightly negative in relation to the room, in order to provide a completely isolated atmosphere for the operator.

3.7 Film Coating Defects

3.7.1 Picking and Sticking

Tablets stick to each other or to the pan due to over wetting and during drying at the point of contact. A piece of the film may remain adhered to the pan or to the another tablet, giving a picked appearance.

Cause	Remedy
• Over-wetting of the tablets,	• Reduction in liquid application rate
• under-drying	• Increase in drying air volume and temperature
• Poor tablet quality.	

3.7.2 Blistering

It is local detachment of film from the substrate forming blister.

Cause	Remedy
• Effect of temperature on the strength, elasticity, and adhesion of the film. • Too rapid evaporation of solvent	• Use mild drying condition.

3.7.3 Chipping

It is a defect where the film becomes chipped and dented, usually at the edges of the tablet.

Cause	Remedy
• High degree of attrition associated with the coating process.	• Increase hardness of the film by increasing the molecular weight grade of polymer.

3.7.4 Cratering

This is the defect of film coating whereby volcanic-like craters appear exposing the tablet surface.

Cause	Remedy
• Inefficient drying.	• Use efficient and optimum drying conditions.
• Higher rate of application of coating solution.	• Increase viscosity of coating solution to decrease spray application rate.

3.7.5 Twinning

Twinning is the term used for two tablets that stick together, and it's a common problem with capsule shaped tablets (Caplets).

Cause	Remedy
• Inefficient drying.	• Use optimum and efficient drying conditions or increase the inlet air temperature.
• Higher rate of application of coating solution	• Decrease the spray rate or increasing the pan speed. • Reducing the

3.7.6 Hazing and Dull Film

It is a defect where coating becomes dull immediately or after prolonged storage at high temperatures.

Cause	Remedy
• High concentration and low molecular weight of plasticizer • High coating temperature • Tablets exposed to higher humidity condition.	• Decrease plasticizer concentration and increase molecular weight of plasticizer. • Decrease the drying air temperature

3.7.7 Colour Variation

A defect which involves variation in colour of the film.

Cause	Remedy
• Improper mixing, • Uneven spray pattern • Insufficient coating • Migration of soluble dyes plasticizers and other additives during drying.	• Reformulation with different plasticizers and additives or use mild drying conditions.

3.7.8 Bridging and Filling

This occurs when the coating film shrinks and pulls away from the sharp corners of an intagliations or bisects and fills in the lettering or logo on the tablet.

Cause	Remedy
• Improper application of the solution • Poor design of the tablet embossing • High coating viscosity • High percentage of solids in the solution • Improper atomization	• Use spray nozzle capable of finer atomization. • Reduce viscosity • Change emboss design

3.7.9 Orange Peel/Roughness

It is surface defect resulting in the film being rough and non-glossy. Appearance is similar to that of an orange. Inadequate spreading of the coating solution before drying gives orange peel effect on the coating.

Causes	Remedy
• Rapid drying • High solution viscosity	• Use mild drying conditions • Use additional solvents to decrease viscosity of solution.

3.7.10 Cracking

Cracking is seen when internal stresses in the film exceeds tensile strength of the film. This is common with higher molecular weight polymers or polymeric blends. So use lower molecular weight polymers or polymeric blends.

Cause	Remedy
• Use of higher molecular weight polymers or polymeric blends.	• Use lower molecular weight polymers or polymeric blends.
	• Adjust plasticizer type and concentration.

3.8   Quality Control

After coating, tablet must be inspected and tested for appearance and performance. Inspection includes check for colour variation, size, appearance and permanent physical defects which may affect performance of the products which include.

Evaluation Parameters:

1. Water vapour permeability
2. Film tensile strength
3. Coated tablet evaluations
   - Adhesion test with tensile-strength tester
   - Diametric crushing strength of coated tablet
   - Film surface roughness
   - Hardness
   - Colour uniformity.

In process quality control

- Weight of tablet
- Crushing strength
- Tablet thickness
- Disintegration time
- Friability
- *In-Vitro* dissolution studies.

Water vapor permeability tests are used to evaluate the effectiveness of a film coating as a barrier to water. Several variables affects water vapor permeability, including film composition, film thickness, and film preparation technique. A tensile test consists of a free film strip that is placed between 2 grips and then stretched at a constant rate until the film fractures. The force and displacement values are recorded during the test and these data are converted to stress and strain.

Most of the above mentioned tests are performed in the same way as they are done for the tablets, with a highlight on the disintegration time as coating is mostly done to increase the time of disintegration.

3.9 Recent Advancements in Coating Techniques

3.9.1 Compressed Coating

It is a dry process of coating, which involves in the compression of granular material around an already pre-formed core (Tablet). It is mainly used to separate incompatible ingredients and also for dual release pattern. This type of coating requires a specialized tablet machine.

3.9.2 Laminate Coating

Laminated coating provides multiple layers for incorporation of medicament.

- *Repeat-action tablet:* In this tablet a portion of the drug is kept in outer coating layer.

- *Enteric tablet:* In this system, one drug is released in gastric region while another in intestinal region.

- *Buccal-swallow tablet:* In this type of tablet first drug is administered sublingually, and after the release of flavour from the inner core, the same may be swallowed as a normal peroral tablet.

3.9.3 Dip Coating

Coating is applied to the tablet cores by dipping them into the coating liquid (waxes and hot melts). The wet tablets are allowed to dry in a conventional manner in coating pan. Alternative dipping and drying steps may be repeated several times to obtain the desired coating. This process lacks the speed, versatility, and reliability of spray-coating techniques.

3.9.4 Vacuum Film Coating

Vacuum film coating employs a specially designed baffled pan which is hot water jacketed, and sealed to achieve a vacuum system. The tablets are placed in the sealed pan, and the air in the pan is displaced by nitrogen before the desired vacuum level is obtained. The coating solution is then applied with airless spray system. The evaporation is caused by the heated pan, and the vapour is removed by the vacuum system. Organic solvent can be effectively used with this coating system with minimum environmental or safety concerns.

3.9.5 Electrostatic Dry Powder Coating

Electrostatic coating is an efficient method of applying coating to conductive substrates. In this, an ionic charge is imparted to the core and an opposite charge to the coating material. The principle of electrostatic powder coating involves spraying of a mixture of finely grounded particles and polymers onto a substrate surface without using any solvent and then heating the substrate for curing on oven until the powder mixture is fused into film (Figure 3.7).

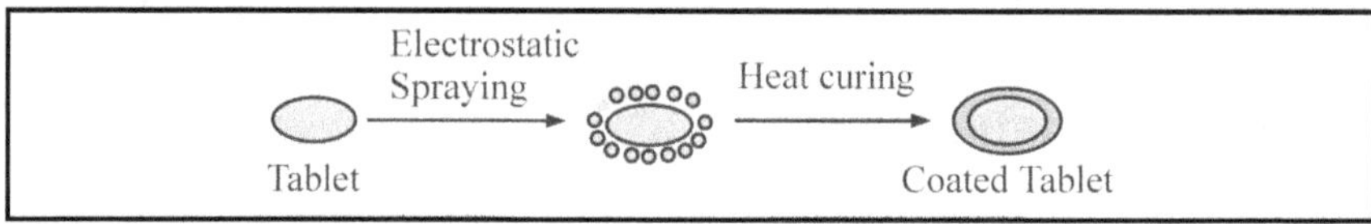

FIGURE 3.7 Electrostatic dry coating.

3.9.6 Magnetically Assisted Impaction Coating (MAIC)

There are several unique features of magnetically assisted impaction coating (MAIC) that make it advantageous as a dry particle coating device. Mechanism of coating in the MAIC process is:

(a) Excitation of magnetic particle

(b) De-agglomeration of guest particles

(c) Shearing and spreading of guest particles on the surface of the host particles

(d) Magnetic–host–host particle interaction

(e) Magnetic–host–wall interaction

(f) Formation of coated products as shown in Figure 3.8.

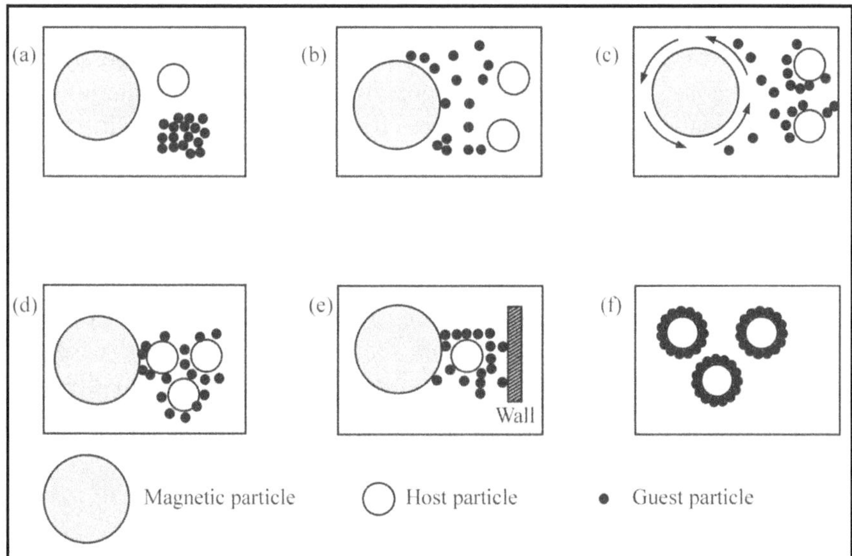

FIGURE 3.8 Mechanism of coating in the MAIC process.

The MAIC can coat soft organic host and guest particles without causing major changes in the material shape and size. There is some heat generated on a microscopic level due to the collisions of particles, there is negligible heat generation on a macroscopic level and hence no increase in temperature of the material during processing by MAIC (Figure 3.9). The device can be operated both as a batch and continuous system making it versatile in the amount of material it can process. This process offers advantage when dealing with temperature sensitive pharmaceuticals.

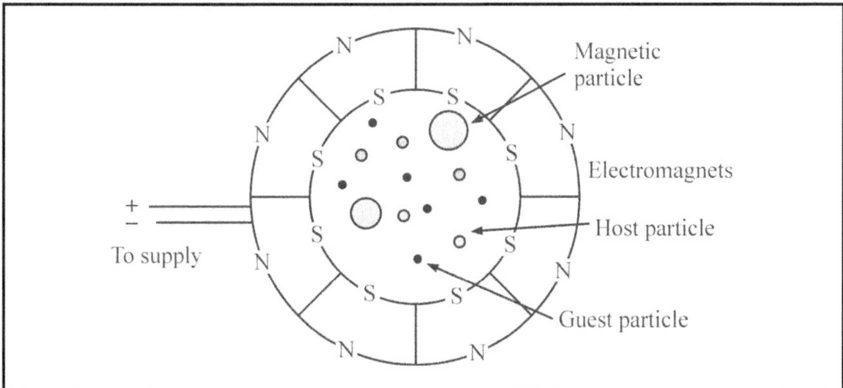

FIGURE 3.9 Schematic diagram of MAIC.

3.9.7 Supercritical Fluid Coating

Coatings of thin films onto solid particle has been achieved by *in-situ* simultaneous nucleation and deposition of dissolved material out of supercritical fluid, resultant film formation on the solid particles suspended in the supercritical fluid, and subsequent thermal conditioning of the coating in the particles.

3.9.8 Opadry® Coating

It is a single composition containing polymer, plasticizer and colourants in a dry concentrate. It provides excellent film forming capabilities including sharp logo definition, high tensile strength and good adhesion properties

4   Capsules

4.1   Introduction

Capsules are solid unit dosage forms in which the medication is contained within an inert, tasteless, gelatin shell and are intended to be taken orally by swallowing them intact or may be administered rectally or vaginally. They are convenient means of dispensing solids, semi-solids, and liquids. Capsules may be hard and soft depending on their composition. The hard capsule consists of two pieces, a smaller cap, which fits over the open end of the longer piece, called the body. The soft gelatin capsule is also called as one-piece encapsulation.

4.1.1   Advantages of Capsules

- Easy to swallow due to slippery nature.
- Elegance, easy to use.
- Mask the taste and odor of unpleasant drugs.
- Fewer adjuncts are required when compare to tablets.
- Easy to handle and transport.

4.1.2   Disadvantages of Capsules

- Hygroscopic drugs, which absorb water from the capsule shell making it brittle, are not suitable for filling into capsules.
- The concentrated solutions which require previous dilution are unsuitable for capsules because if administered as such may lead to irritation of stomach.
- Very soluble materials, such as bromides or iodides are not suitable to dispense in capsules, as the rapid release of such materials may cause gastric irritation.
- Not tamper proof.

4.2   Manufacturing of Hard Gelatin Capsules

The raw materials used in the manufacture of both hard and soft gelatin capsules are similar. Both contain gelatin, water, colourants, certified dyes, plasticizers and preservatives.

4.2.1 Gelatin

Gelatin is a heterogeneous product obtained by irreversible hydrolytic extraction of treated animal collagen, which is obtained from animal bones, white connective tissues, and the skin. It is a translucent, vitreous brittle solid, colorless or slightly yellow, tasteless and odorless. Gelatin contains 8-13% moisture and has a relative density of 1.3-1.4. Gelatin is soluble in aqueous solutions of polyhydric alcohols such as glycerol and propylene glycol. Gelatin in solution is amphoteric, capable of acting either as an acid or as a base. Gelatin has been the raw material of choice because of the ability of a solution to gel to form a solid at a temperature just above ambient temperate conditions, which enables a homogeneous film to be formed rapidly on a mould pin. Gelatin possesses the following basic properties:

- Inert and non-toxic.
- It is readily soluble in biological fluids at body temperature.
- It is good film-forming material, producing a strong flexible film.
- The Gelatin films are homogeneous in structure, and have high strength.

Disadvantage with using gelatin for hard capsules is that it has a high moisture content and also undergoes a cross linking reaction that reduces its solubility. It is stable when dry but is subject to microbial decomposition in presence of moisture.

Types of Gelatin

Gelatin derived from an acid-treated precursor is known as Type A and which is derived from an alkali-treated process is known as Type B.

- Type A gelatin is derived from an acid-treated precursor and exhibits an isoelectric point in the region of pH 7.0-9.0.
- Type B gelatin is obtained from an alkali-treated precursor and has its isoelectric point in the region of pH 4.8-5.0.

Capsules may be made from either type of gelatin, but mostly a mixture of both types is preferable considering availability and cost. Blends of bone and pork skin gelatins of relatively high strength are normally used for hard capsule production. The bone gelatin produces a tough and firm film, but tends to be hazy and brittle. The pork skin gelatin provides plasticity and clarity to the blend; reducing haze or cloudiness in the finished capsule. The General specification of Gelatin A and B are given in Table 4.1

On heating Gelatin melts and solidifies when cooled again. Together with water it forms a semi-solid colloidal gel.

TABLE 4.1

A hard capsule gelatin specification

Characteristics	Type A	Type B
Gel strength	240-300	200-250
Viscosity (milli poise)	44-55	45-60
pH	4.5-5.5	5.3-6.5

Production of Gelatin

The principal raw materials used in gelatin production are cattle bones, cattle hides, and pork skins. The raw materials are prepared by different curing, acid, and alkali processes which are employed to extract the dried collagen hydrolysate. The entire process takes several weeks. Both of these classes of capsules are made from gelling agents like gelatin, plant polysaccharides or their derivatives like carrageenan and modified forms of starch and cellulose. Other additives like plasticizers such as glycerine or sorbitol to decrease the capsule's hardness, colouring agents, preservatives, disintegrants, lubricants is a process and not an additive are used.

The flow chart for gelatin production has been shown in Figure 4.1.

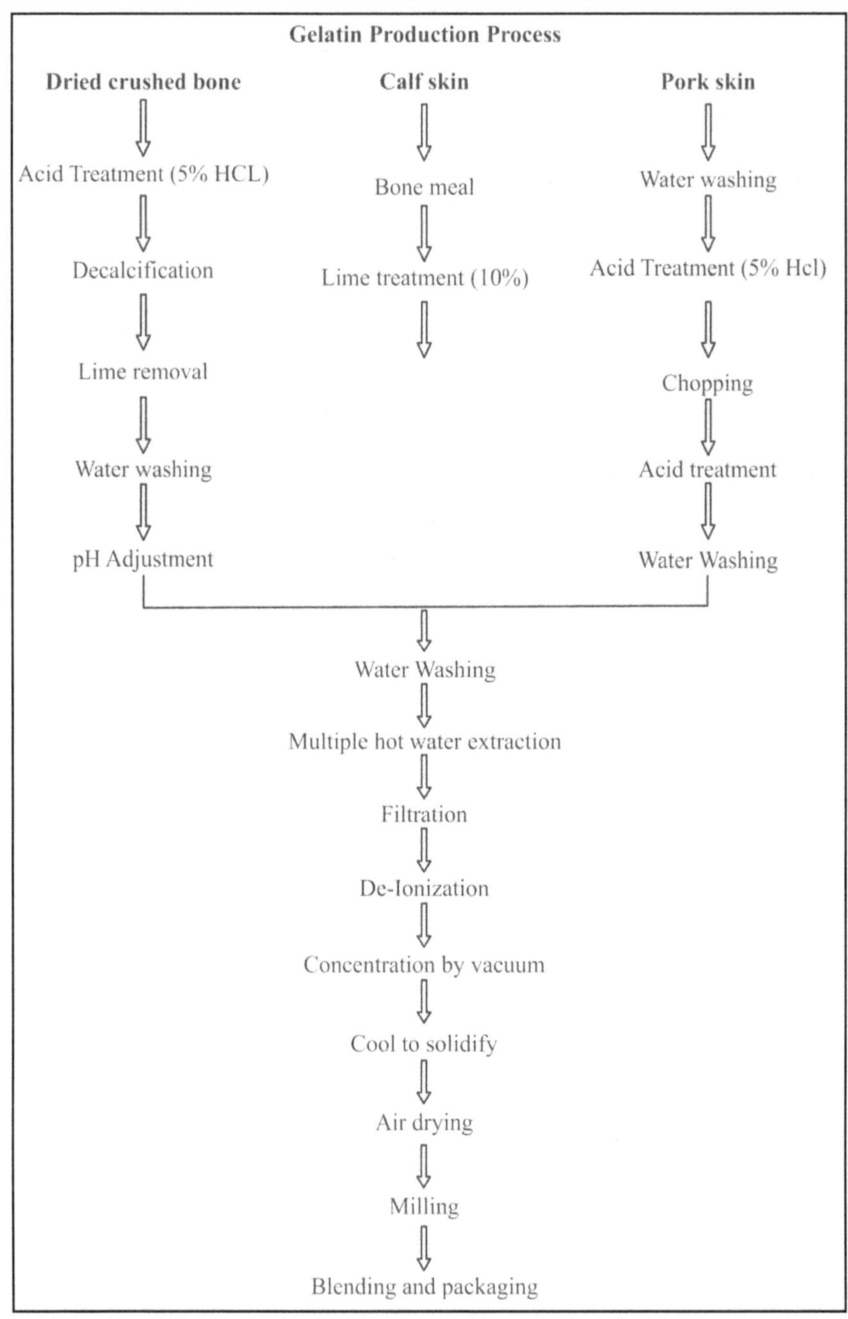

FIGURE 4.1 Flow chart for gelatin production.

4.2.2 Plasticizers

The plasticizers used are glycerol, sorbitol, propylene glycol, sucrose etc. The exact proportions of gelatin and plasticizers have to be determined on the basis of the use of capsules and their storage conditions.

4.2.3 Colourants

Colourants are used to identify the product and to improve patient compliance. Commonly soluble synthetic dyes (coal tar) and insoluble pigments are used. Commonly iron-oxide is used.

4.2.4 Opacifying Agents

They are used to make shell opaque. Opaque capsules are used to provide protection against light and to conceal the contents e.g., titanium-dioxide.

4.2.5 Preservatives

Preservatives are added to the gelatin and colorant solutions to reduce the growth of micro-organisms *e.g.*, bisulfite or metabisulfite, sorbic acid or the methyl propyl esters of parahydroxy-benzoic acid and organic acids like benzoic and propanoic acids.

4.2.6 Wetting Agent

To ensure that the lubricated metal moulds are uniformly covered when dipped into the gelatin solution. *e.g.*, Surfactants.

4.3   Method of Production of Hard Gelatin Capsule Shells

Hard gelatin capsule shells are manufactured in two sections, the body and the shorter cap. The method commonly used for capsule production consists of mechanisms for dipping, spinning, drying, stripping, trimming, and joining the capsules.

1. *Dipping*: One hundred and fifty pairs of stainless steel pins are dipped into the gelatin solution reservoir of carefully controlled viscosity to form caps and bodies simultaneously.

2. *Spinning*: The pins are rotated to uniformly distribute the gelatin, during which time the gelatin may be set or gelled by a blast of cool air

3. ***Drying***: The pins are moved through a series of controlled air drying kilns for the gradual precise and controlled removal of water

4. ***Stripping***: Now the capsules are stripped from the pins with the help of the bronze jaws

5. ***Trimming***: After stripping, the excess of length is trimmed with the help of stationary knives.

6. ***Joining***: The cap and body sections are joined and ejected from the machine. The entire cycle of the machine lasts approximately 45 min.

Thickness of the capsule wall is controlled by:

- Viscosity of the gelatin solution
- The speed and time of dipping
- Mould pin dimensions
- Precise drying
- Cut lengths

The in-process quality controls include periodic monitoring, and adjustment when required, of film thickness, cut lengths of cap and body, colour, and moisture content.

4.3.1 Types of Materials for Filling into Hard Gelatin Capsules

1. ***Dry solids***: Powders, pellets, granules or tablets.
2. ***Semisolids***: Suspensions or pastes.
3. ***Liquids***: Non-aqueous liquids.

4.3.2 Capsule Size

Hard-shell capsule sizes range from no. 5, (the smallest) to 000, which is the largest used for veterinary sizes. However, size No. 00 generally is the largest size acceptable to human patients.

4.3.3 Determinations of Capsule Fill Weight

Capsule fill weight = tapped bulk density of formulation × capsule volume

Physical specification for Hard gelatin capsules are as shown in Table 4.2.

TABLE 4.2

Physical specifications for hard gelatin capsule

Size	Outer diameter (mm)	Height or Locked length (mm)	Actual volume (mL)	Typical fill weights (mg) of Powder density 0.70 g/mL
000	9.91	26.14	1.40	960
00	8.53	23.30	0.95	665
0	7.65	21.70	0.68	475
1	6.91	19.40	0.50	350
2	6.35	18.00	0.37	260
3	5.82	15.90	0.30	210
4	5.31	14.30	0.21	145
5	4.91	11.10	0.13	90

4.3.4 Filling of Hard Gelatin Capsules

Hard-shell capsules typically are filled with powder, beads, granules, tablets, semisolids or liquids also may be filled into hard-shell capsules; however, when the latter are encapsulated, one of the sealing techniques must be employed to prevent leakage. Excipients generally used are;

4.3.4.1 Diluents

Diluents are the excipients that are usually present in the greatest concentration in a formulation and they make up the necessary bulk when the quantity of the active ingredient is insufficient to make up the required bulk e.g. Lactose, mannitol, maize starch, calcium sulfate etc.

4.3.4.2 Lubricants and Glidants

These are the excipients which reduce powder to metal adhesion and promote flow properties *e.g.*: magnesium stearate, stearic acid, talc.

4.3.4.3 Wetting Agents

Wetting agents improve water penetration for poorly soluble drugs *e.g.*: Sodium lauryl sulphate, tween 80.

4.3.5 Hand Filling Gelatin Capsule Machine

A hand operated filling machine as shown in Figure 4.2 consists of the following parts:

1. A bed with 200-300 holes
2. A capsule loading tray
3. A powder tray
4. A pin plate having 200 or 300 pins corresponding to the number of holes in the bed and capsule loading tray
5. A lever
6. A handle
7. A plate fitted with rubber top.

In hard gelatin capsule filling operations, the body and cap the of the shell are separated prior to dosing. Machines employing various dosing principles may be employed to fill powders into hard-shell capsules; however, most fully automatic machines form powder plugs by compression and eject them into empty capsule bodies.

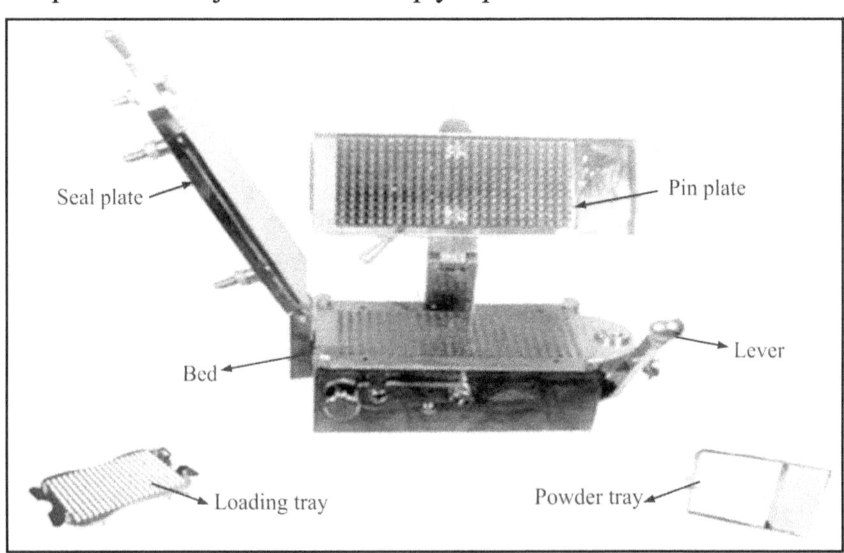

FIGURE 4.2 Hand operated hard gelatin capsule filling machine.

1. ***Working:*** The empty capsules are filled into the loading tray, which is then placed over the bed. By opening the handle, the

bodies of the capsules are locked and caps separated in the loading tray itself, which is then removed by operating the liver. The weighed amount of the drug to be filled in the capsules is placed in powder tray already kept in position over the bed. Spread the powder with the help of a powder spreader so as to fill the bodies of the capsules uniformly. Collect excess of the powder on the platform of the powder tray. Lower the pin plate and move it downward so as to press the powder in the bodies. Remove the powder tray and place the caps holding tray in position. Press the caps with the help of plate with rubber top and operate the lever to unlock the cap and body of the capsules. Remove the loading tray and collect the filled capsules in a tray. With 200-hole machine about 5000 capsules can be filled per hour and with 300-hole machine 7500 capsules can be filled per hour.

On large-scale manufacturing, various types of semi automatic and automatic machines are used. They operate on the same principle as manual filling, namely the caps are removed, powder filled in the bodies, caps replaced, and filled capsules are ejected out. With automatic capsule filling machines, powders or granulated products can be filled into hard gelatin capsules. With accessory equipment, pellets or tablets along with powders can be filled into the capsules.

2. *Capsule filling devices*: A number of different manually operated capsule filling devices are commercially available for filling up to 50 or 100 capsules at a time. The method of using these machines requires a careful determination of the capsule formulation. Machine automatically separate the cap from the empty capsules, fill the bodies, scrape off the excess powder, replace the caps, seal the capsules as desired and clean the outside of the filled capsule. The process flow chart for the automated filling machine is shown in Figure 4.3 figure here.

The dosing systems can be divided into two groups:

Dependent: These are the dosing systems that use the capsule body directly to measure the powder. Uniformity of fill weight can only be achieved if the capsule is filled completely. *E.g.*: Auger filling.

Independent: These are the dosing systems where the powder is measured independently of the body in a special measuring device. Weight uniformity is not dependent on filling the body completely. With this system the capsules can be partly filled. *E.g.*: Dosator. An illustration of dosator principle is shown in Figure 4.4.

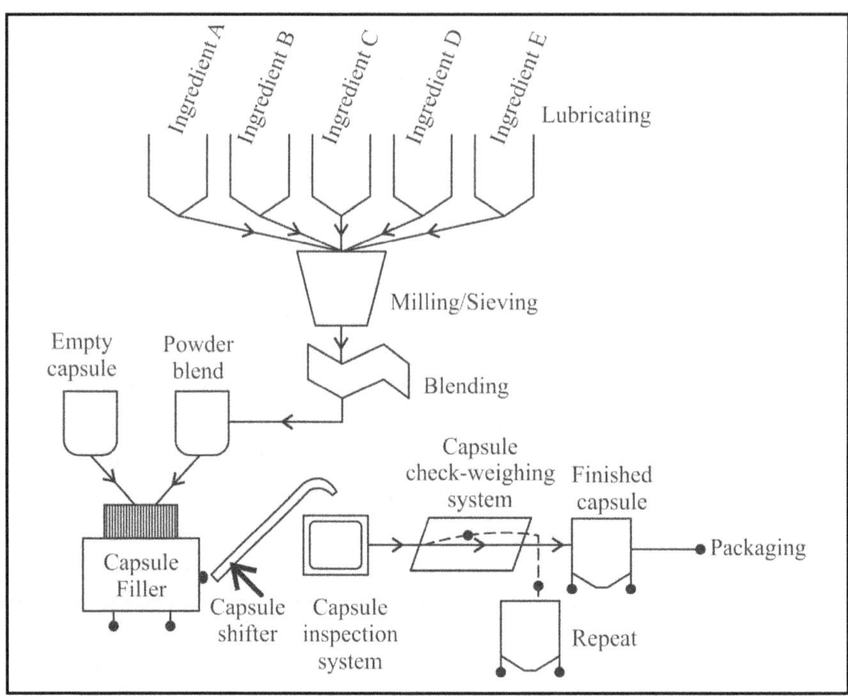

FIGURE 4.3 Process flow diagram for automated capsule filling.

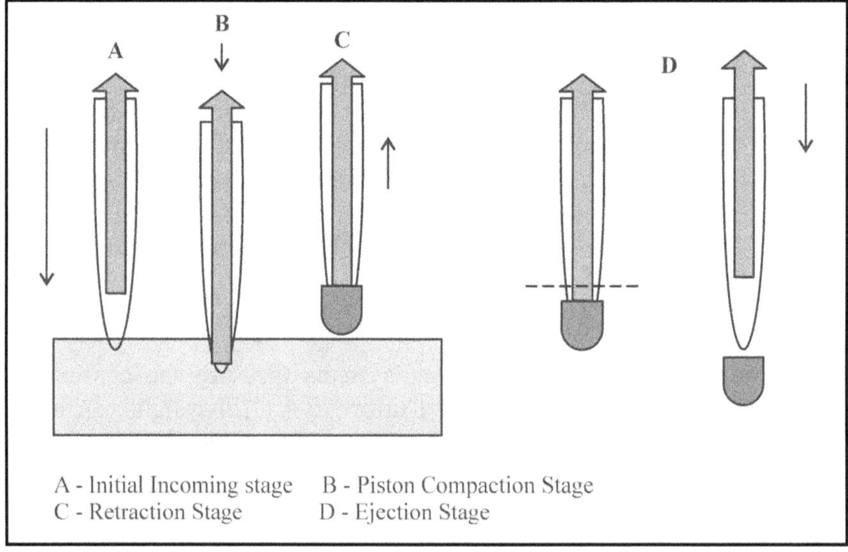

FIGURE 4.4 Dosator Capsule filling.

4.3.6 Cleaning and Polishing

1. *Pan polishing*: Accela cota coting pan is used to dust and polish capsule. A polyurethane or cheese liner cloth is used to trap the removed dust and to impart gloss.

2. *Cloth dusting*: Cloth impregnated with or without oil is used.

3. *Brushing*: Capsules are fed under rotating soft brushes which removes dust.

4.4 Soft Gelatin Capsules

A soft gel (a soft gelatine capsule) is a solid capsule (outer shell) which consists of a liquid or semi-solid inside a one-piece gelatin shell. Soft gelatin capsules are one-piece and hermetically sealed to enclose a liquid or semi-liquid fill. Gelatin soft capsules are made from gelatin and water but with the addition of a polyhydric alcohol, such as glycerol or sorbitol, to make them flexible. Soft capsules are primarily used for oils and for active ingredients that are dissolved or suspended in oil.

They are available in variety of shapes and sizes as:

- Spherical – 0.05-5 mL
- Ovoid – 0.05-7 mL
- Cylindrical – 0.15-25 mL
- Tubes – 0.5-0 mL
- Pear shaped – 0.3-5 mL

They are most suitable for liquids and semisolids and are widely used, in spherical and ovoid forms for vitamin preparations such as cod liver oil, vitamins A and D and multiple vitamins. The specification of soft gels is as shown in Table 4.3.

TABLE 4.3

A soft capsule gelatin specification

Characteristics	Type A	Type B
Gel strength	150-200	125-175
Viscosity (millipoise)	25-35	30-45
pH	4.5-5.5	5.3-6.5

Advantages of soft gel capsules

1. Ease of use, easy to swallow, no taste.
2. Accommodates a wide variety of compounds filled as a semisolid, liquid, gel or paste.
3. Available in wide variety of colors, shapes and sizes.
4. Immediate or delayed drug delivery can be used to improve bioavailability.
5. Wide variety of application as an oral, topical, ophthalmic, and otic dosage form.
6. Unit dose delivery, tamper proof.

Disadvantages of soft gel capsules

1. Requires specialized manufacturing equipment.
2. Highly sensitive to temperature and humidity.
3. Additional quality control measures may be required.

There are three primary types of inner fill materials, which are:

1. ***Oily liquid***: Oily active liquid ingredients such as, cod liver oil, clofibrate etc.
   - Water miscible volatile and non-volatile liquid such as vegetable and aromatic oil, hydrocarbons, ethers, esters, alcohols, and organic acids.
   - Water miscible non volatile liquids such as polyethylene glycols
   - Water miscible liquid such as propylene glycol and isopropyl alcohol
2. ***Solutions***: Active ingredients dissolved in a solvent should be air free, homogenous, and solvent, which does not degrade or solubilize the gelatin shell.
3. ***Suspension fills***: These suspension fills have active ingredients dispersed in a solvent. Suspensions can accommodate about 30% solids and should flow by gravity at room temperature. Suspended solids must be smaller than 80-mesh mill or homogenize before filling to prevent needles from clogging during filling.

The formulation of suspensions for capsulation follows the basic concepts of suspension technology. Formulation techniques, however, can be carried out depending on the drug substance, the desired flow characteristics, the physical or ingredient stability problems, or the biopharmaceutical properties desired. In the formulation of suspensions for soft gelatin encapsulation, certain basic information must be developed to determine minimum capsule size.

Base adsorption of solids to be suspended in soft gelatin capsules

Base adsorption of solid is used to determine the size of capsule. It is expressed as the number of grams of liquid base required to produce a consultable mixture when mixed with one gram of solid(s). The base adsorption of a solid is influenced by such factors such as the solids particle size and shape, its physical state, its density, its moisture content, and its lipophilic or hydrophilic nature. In the determination of base adsorption, the solid(s) must be completely wetted by the liquid base.

A practical procedure for determining base adsorption and for judging the adequate fluidity of a mixture is as follows:

Weigh a defined amount of the solid (40 g is convenient) into a 150 ml tarred beaker. In a separate 150 ml tarred beaker, place about 100 g of the solid base. Add small increments of the liquid base to the solid, and using a spatula, stir the base into the solid after each addition until the solid is thoroughly wetted and uniformly coated with the base. This should produce a mixture that has a soft ointment like consistency. Continue to add liquid and stir until the mixture flows steadily from the spatula blade when held at a 45° angle above the mixture.

The base adsorption is obtained by means of the following formula

$$\text{Base Adsorption} = \frac{\text{Weight of the base}}{\text{Weight of the solid}} \qquad \text{.... (4.1)}$$

The base adsorption is used to determine the "minim per gram" factor (M/g) of the solid(s). The minim per gram factor is the volume in minims that is occupied by one gram (S) of the solid plus the weight of the liquid base (BA) required to make a capsulatable mixture. The minimum per gram factor is calculated by dividing the weight of the base plus the gram of solid base (BA+ S) by the weight of the mixture (W) per cubic centimeter or 16.23 minims (V).

$$(BA + S) \times \frac{V}{W} = \frac{M}{g} \qquad \text{.... (4.2)}$$

Thus lower the base adsorption of the solid (s) and higher the density of the mixture, the smaller the capsule will be. This also indicates the importance of establishing specifications for the control of those physical properties of a solid mentioned previously that can affect its base adsorption.

The final formulation of a suspension invariably requires a suspending agent to prevent the settling of the solids and to maintain homogeneity prior to, during, and after capsulation. For hydrophobic bases, waxes and for hydrophilic ones, Poly Ethylene Glycol 4000, Poly Ethylene Glycol 6000 are generally used. Sometimes incorporation of wetting agents such as soy lecithin becomes necessary when the solids are not properly wetted by the base.

4.4.1 Manufacturing of Soft Gelatin Capsules

4.4.1.1 Rotary Capsule Machine

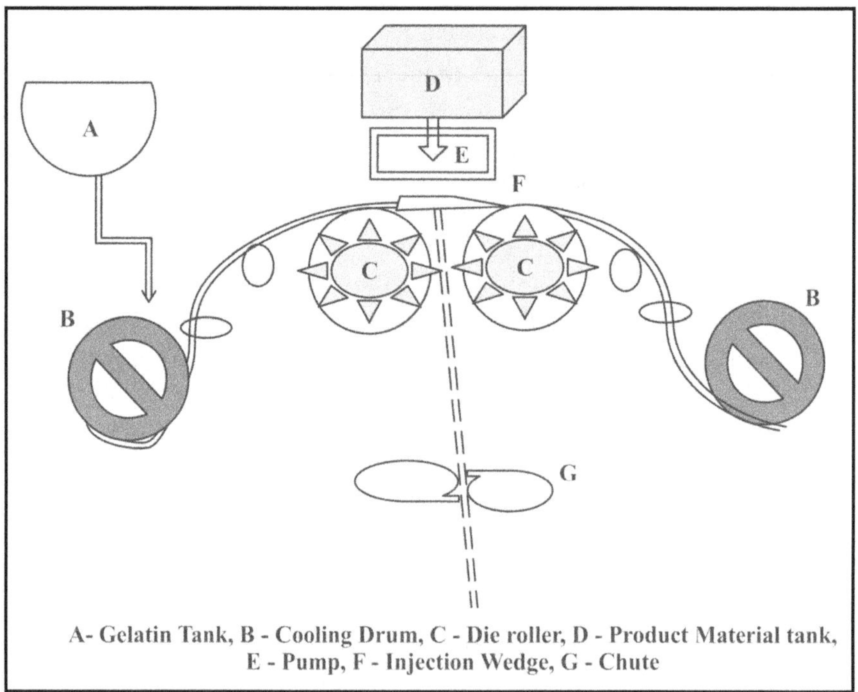

A- Gelatin Tank, B - Cooling Drum, C - Die roller, D - Product Material tank, E - Pump, F - Injection Wedge, G - Chute

FIGURE 4.5 Rotary capsule machine.

Soft shell capsules are both formed, filled, and sealed in the same machine; typically, this is a rotary die process, although a plate process or reciprocating die process also may be employed. This machine consists of two, cylinders in each of which half-moulds are cut. These cylinders rotate in contrary direction. Two ribbons of gelatin are fed between the rollers and, just before the opposing rollers meet, jets of medicament press the gelatin ribbon into the moulds, filling each half. The moment of pressure follows, immediately sealing the two halves together to form a capsule. An automated soft gelatin encapsulation machine is shown in Figure 4.5.

4.4.1.2 Seamless Gelatin Capsules

Soft-shell capsules also may be manufactured in a bubble process that forms seamless spherical capsules. With suitable equipment, powders and other dry solids can also be filled into soft-shell capsules. Another method of making soft gelatin capsules takes advantage of the phenomenon of drop formation. The essential part of the apparatus consists of two concentric tubes. Through the inner tube flows the medicament and, through the surrounding outer tube, the gelatin solution. The medicament, therefore, issues from the tube surrounded by gelatin and forming a spherical drop. This is ensured by allowing the drop to form in liquid paraffin in which the gelatin is insoluble. Regular induced pulsations cause drops of the correct size to be formed, and a temperature of 4°C ensures that the gelatin shell is rapidly congealed. The capsules are subsequently degreased and dried.

4.4.2 Formulation of Soft Gelatin Capsules

1. *Gelatin shell formulation*: Typical soft gelatin capsules are made up of gelatin, plasticizer, and materials that impart the desired appearance (colorants and/or opacifiers), and sometimes flavors.

2. *Plasticizers*: These are used to make the softgel shell elastic and pliable. They usually account for 20-30%. The most common plasticizers used in softgels are glycerin, sorbitol and propylene glycol are used frequently often in combination with glycerol. Plasticizers are selected on the basis of their compatibility with the fill formulation, ease of processing, and the desired properties of the final soft gel, including hardness, appearance, handling characteristics and physical stability. The ratio by weight of dry plasticizer to dry gelatin determines the hardness of the gelatin shell.

3. *Water*: The other essential component of the soft gel shell is water. Water usually accounts for 30-40 % of the wet gel formulation and its presence is important to ensure proper processing during gel preparation and softgel encapsulation.

4. *Colourants/opacifiers*: Colourants (soluble dyes, or insoluble pigments or lakes) and opacifiers are typically used in the wet gel formulation. Colourants can be either synthetic or natural, and are used to impart the desired shell color for product identification. An opacifier, usually titanium dioxide may be added to produce an opaque shell when the fill formulation is a suspension, or to prevent photo degradation of light-sensitive fill ingredients. Titanium dioxide can either be used alone to produce a white opaque shell or in combination with pigments to produce a colored opaque shell.

4.5   Quality Control of Capsules

Quality control should be carried out during all stages of manufacturing operation, which is the primary requirement of good manufacturing practices. The hard and soft gelatin capsules should be subjected to following tests for their standardization.

1. Shape and size
2. Colour
3. Uniformity of mass for single-dose preparations
4. Content Uniformity
5. Thickness of capsule shell
6. Leaking test for semi-solid and liquid ingredients from soft capsules
7. Disintegration tests
8. Weight variation test

4.5.1 Weight Variation

Weigh 20 intact capsules individually, and calculate the average mass. The mass of each capsule should be within ±10% of the average mass. If all the capsules do not fall within these limits, weigh 20 capsules again, taking care to preserve the identity of each capsule, and remove the contents as completely as possible. Wash the shell with ether or some other suitable solvent and allow it to stand until the odour of the solvent is no longer perceptible. Other means, such as a jet of compressed air, may be used to remove the contents.

Weigh the emptied shells individually and calculate for each capsule the net mass of its contents by subtracting the mass of the shell from the gross mass. Determine the average net content from the sum of the individual net masses. Then determine the difference between each individual net content and the average net content. Deviation of individual net mass from the average net mass should not exceed the limits given below.

TABLE 4.4

Limit of capsule for weight variation test

Net mass of capsule contents	% Deviation	Number of capsules from the selected (20)
less than 300 mg	± 10.0	minimum 18
	± 20.0	maximum 2
300 mg and over	± 7.5	minimum 18
	± 15.0	maximum 2

4.5.2 Content Uniformity

Each single unit contains within ± 15% of the average amount of active ingredient. However, if up to three individual units deviate by more than ± 15% but are within ± 25% of the average amount of the active ingredient, examine a further 20 units drawn from the same original sample as the first 10 units. The preparation under test complies only if the amount of active ingredient found in no more than three out of 30 units deviates by more than ± 15% of the average amount. None deviates by more than ± 25% of the average amount.

4.5.3 Disintegration

Tablet disintegration test apparatus is used to perform the disintegration test of capsules also. According to USP, place one dosage unit in each of the tubes of the basket with water or any other specified medium (depends on individual monograph) maintained at 37 ±2 °C. The capsules pass the test if no residue of drug or other fragments of shell remains on No.10 mesh screen of the tubes. If 1 or 2 capsules fail, the test should be repeated on additional of 12 capsules. Then, not fewer than 16 of the total 18 capsules tested should disintegrate completely.

4.5.4 Dissolution

Place each of the capsules in the apparatus 1, excluding air bubbles from the surface of the capsule. Operate immediately at specified rate within specified dissolution medium at 37 ± 0.5 °C. Aliquots should be withdrawn at specified time points mentioned in individual monograph.

The requirements are met if the quantity of active ingredients dissolved confirms the following:

1. ***At stage* 1 (S1):** When 6 capsules are tested, amount of each of the dissolved content should not be less than ± 5% of the mentioned in monograph.

2. ***At stage* 2 (S2):** When 6 capsules are tested, the average of 12 (both from step 1 and 2) should be equal to or greater than 15% and no capsule should be less than 15%.

3. ***At stage* 3 (S3):** When 12 capsules are tested, the average of 24 capsules (all 1, 2 and 3 steps) should be equal to or greater than the amount mentioned in the monograph, not more than two units should be less than 15% and no units should be less than 25%.

4.5.5 Capsule Stability

Unprotected soft capsules rapidly reach equilibrium with the atmospheric conditions under which they are stored. The physical stability of soft gelatin capsules is associated primarily with the pick-up or loss of water by the capsule shell. If these are prevented by proper packaging, the above control capsule should have satisfactory physical stability at temperature ranging from just above freezing to as high as 60 °C, for the unprotected control capsule, low humidities (less than 20% RH), low temperature (less than 2 °C) and high temperatures (greater than 38 °C) or combinations of these conditions have only transient effects. The total moisture content of the capsule shell, at equilibrium with any given relative humidity within a reasonable temperature range, should closely approximate the sum of the moisture content of the glycerin and the gelatin when held separately at the stated conditions. Capsules containing water-soluble or miscible liquid bases may be affected to a greater extent than oil-based capsules, owing to the residual moisture in the capsule content and to the dynamic relationship existing between capsule shell and capsule fill during the drying process. Temperate and Humidity have a detrimental effect on the various properties of capsules shell as depicted in Table 4.5

TABLE 4.5

Effect of temperature and humidity on capsule shell

Temperature	Humidity	Effect on capsule shell
21-24 °C	60%	Capsules become softer, tackier and bloated
Greater than 24 °C	Greater than 45%	More rapid and pronounced effects – unprotected capsules melt and fuse together

4.5.5.1 Accelerated Physical Stability Tests

The capsule manufacturers routinely conduct accelerated physical stability tests on all new capsule products as an integral part of the product development program. The following tests have proved adequate for determining the effect of the capsule shell content on the gelatin shell. The tests are strictly relevant to the integrity of the gelatin shell and should not be confused as stability tests for the active ingredients in the capsule content. The results of such tests are used as a guide for the reformulation of the capsule content or the capsule shell, or for the selection of the proper retail package. The test conditions for such accelerated physical stability conditions are shown in table.

TABLE 4.6

Test conditions for accelerated physical stability tests for capsule dosage forms

Test Conditions	Observation
80% Relative humidity at room temperature in an open container	Capsules are observed periodically for 2 weeks; both gross and subtle effects of the storage conditions are noted and recorded. The control capsule should not be affected.
40 °C in an open container	
40 °C in a closed container (glass bottle with tight screw-cap)	Except at the 80% RH station.

The capsules at these stations are observed periodically for 2 weeks. Both gross and subtle effects of the storage conditions on the capsule shell are noted and recorded. The control capsule should not be affected except at the 80% RH station, where the capsule would react as described under the effects of high humidity.

4.6   Packaging and Storage of Capsules

The empty capsules should be stored in tight containers until they are filled. Since gelatin is of animal origin and starch is of vegetable origin, capsules made with these materials should be protected from potential sources of microbial contamination.

Capsules should be packed in a well-closed glass or plastic containers and stored in a cool place.

Empty gelatin capsules should be stored at room temperature at constant humidity. High humidity may cause softening of the capsules and low humidity may cause drying and cracking of the capsules. Storage of capsules in glass containers will provide protection not only from extreme humidity but also from dust.

Storage of filled capsules is dependent on the characteristics of the drugs they contain. Semisolid filled hard gelatin capsules should be stored away from excessive heat, which may cause a softening or melting of the contents.

4.7   Recent Advancements in Capsule Formulation

Recent advancements in the field of capsule formulation are broadly categorized as:

- **A. Development in capsule system:** It includes modification of the system to achieve modified release.
- **B. Development in capsule shell:** It includes modification of capsule shell to improve shell property.

PORT Capsule Technology

Programmable oral release technologies (PORT) is a unique coated encapsulated system which provides multiple program release of the drug. Port technologies offer significant flexibility in obtaining unique and desirable release profile to maximize pharmacological and therapeutic effect. *E.g.* Delayed release pseudoephedrine, multiple program release of phenylpropanolamine.

Chew Caps™ / Soft Burst^{Tm}

They are chewable soft gelatin capsules containing a range of flavors. The fill of chew caps has been designed to maximize its taste and mouth feel.

Hydrophilic Sandwich Capsules

It is a simple and time delayed probe capsule, with a capsule inside a capsule, in which the inter capsular space is filled with a layer of hydrophilic polymer (HPMC). This effectively creates a "Hydrophilic Sandwich" between two gelatin capsule. When the outer capsule is dissolved, the sandwich of HPMC forms a gel barrier layer that provides a time delay before the fluid can enter the inner capsule and cause drug release. The time delay is controlled by molecular weight of polymer and inclusion of soluble filler. *E.g.*: Lactose.

Capsule in Capsule Technology

DUOCAP™ is a patented capsule-in-capsule delivery system that is ideally suited for combination or dual release products. This delivery system involves inserting a smaller pre-filled capsule (Liquid, semisolid, powder or pellets) into a larger liquid-filled capsule, offers a broad range of formulation and design options such as, combination and dual release products, Immediate and controlled release options, with sustained, pulsed or delayed release profile.

Press-Fit® & Xpress-Fit™

The Press-Fit® & Xpress-Fit™ Gel caps enrobe caplets with a high-gloss gel cover, that will create a new look and energize sales. The standard Press-Fit® configuration is completely covered by two flexible gel caps. The Xpress-Fit™ design imparts a gap between the two gel caps, enabling the potential for a fast-release dosage form as well as providing a novel appearance.

Delayed Release Capsules

Capsules may be coated, or, more commonly, encapsulated granules may be coated to resist releasing the drug in the gastric fluid of the stomach where a delay is important to alleviate potential problems of drug inactivation or gastric mucosal irritation.

Non Gelatin Capsule Shell

The animal source of gelatin can be a problem for certain patients such as vegetarians or religious or ethnic group. Unmodified gelatin is prone to cross linking when in contact with aldehydes, solubility problems might be expected with certain fill formulations. This drawback could be overcome by using non-gelatin capsule shells are made up of Starch, HPMC, Poly Vinyl Alcohol and Alginate.

5   Microencapsulation

5.1   Introduction

Microencapsulation is a process by which solids, liquids or even gases may be enclosed in microscopic particles forming a thin continuous polymeric coating. A microcapsule is a small sphere surrounded with a uniform thin wall. The material inside the microcapsule is referred as the core or internal phase, whereas the outer coating as a shell. Most microcapsules have diameters between a few micrometers and a few millimetres. The lowest particle size of microcapsules is 1 μm and the largest size is 1mm.

The uniqueness of microencapsulation technique is the smallness of the coated particles and their subsequent use and adaptation to a wide variety of dosage forms.

Classification

Microcapsules can be classified on the basis of morphology as:

1. Mononuclear (microcapsules contain the shell around the core)
2. Polynuclear (capsules have many cores enclosed within the shell)
3. Matrix types (the core material is distributed homogeneously into the shell material)

5.2   Reason of Microencapsulation

- To provide the means of converting liquids to free flowing powders.
- To provide environmental protection to reactive substances.
- To control the release characteristics of drug substance.
- To separate incompatible components for functional reasons

- To alters colloidal and surface properties.

- To mask taste and odour of many drugs and improve patient compliance.

5.3 Applications of Microencapsulation

There are almost limitless applications of microencapsulated material. Microencapsulated materials are utilized in agriculture, pharmaceuticals, foods, cosmetics and fragrances, textiles, paper, paints, coatings, adhesives, printing applications, and is also used in many other industries. As depicted in Figure 5.1.

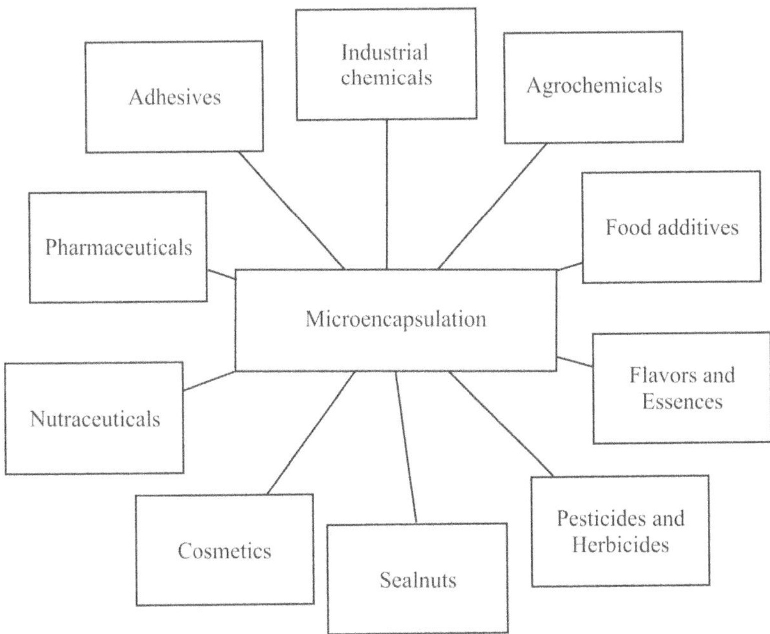

FIGURE 5.1 Application of microencapsulation.

- It provides the means of converting liquids to solids *e.g.*: liquid crystals, Eprazinone.

- Because of the smallness of the particles, drug moieties can be widely distributed throughout the gastrointestinal tract, thus potentially improving drug absorption.

- Altered release characteristics such as sustained release or prolonged action can be attained. *e.g.*: isosorbide dinitrate.

- Taste masking *e.g.*: Acetaminophen, Nitrofurantoin.

- Stabilization against oxidation *e.g.*: Vitamin A palmitate.

- Reduction of volatility *e.g.*: menthol, methyl salicylate.

- Reduced gastric irritation *e.g.*: aspirin.

- Also can be applied in new formulation concepts such as chewable tablets, creams, ointments, aerosols, suppositories and injectables.

5.4 Formulation

Microencapsulation process involves the basic understanding of the general properties of microcapsules such as the nature of core and coating materials, the stability, and release characteristics of the coated materials and the microencapsulation methods.

5.4.1 Core Material

It is the material to be coated which can be either a liquid or a solid. The composition of core material can be varied which include liquid core such as dispersed and /or dissolved materials and solid core which can be a mixture of active constituents and stabilizers, diluents, excipients and release rate retardants or accelerators.

Types of core material and their purpose are shown in table 5.1

Purpose of Encapsulation	Core Material
Taste Masking	Acetaminophene
Reduce gastric irritation	Aspirin
Stabilization (Conversion of Liquid to solids)	Liquid crystals
Oxidative Stabilization	Vitamin A Patmitate
Sustained release	Isosorbide dinitrate, Progesterone
Reduction of Volatility	Methyl saliocylate, camphor
Selective sorption	Activated charcoal

5.4.2 Encapsulation Material

It is the material, which is coated.

Ideal characteristics of coating material:

- Should be capable of forming a film that must be cohesive.
- Should be chemically compatible and non-reactive with the core material.
- Should provide desired coating properties such as strength, flexibility, impermeability, optical properties and stability.

5.5 Types of Encapsulation Materials

(a) *Water Soluble Resins*: Gelatin, Gum Arabic, Starch, Methyl Cellulose, PVP, Hydroxyl propyl methyl cellulose (HPMC), and Polyvinyl Acetate.

(a) *Water Insoluble Resins*: Ethyl cellulose, polyethylene, cellulose nitrate and silicones.

(c) *Waxes and Lipids*: Paraffin, carnauba wax, beeswax, stearic acid, stearyl alcohol.

(d) *Enteric Resins*: Shellac, cellulose acetate phthalate, Zein etc.

Film thickness can be varied depending on:

- Surface area of the material to be encapsulated.
- Physical characteristics of the system.

5.6 Techniques of Microencapsulation

(a) **Chemical Methods**

- Interfacial polymerization
- *In situ* polymerization

(b) Physico-chemical Process

- Coacervation and phase separation.
- Rapid expansion of supercritical fluid
- Gas anti-solvent (GAS) process

(c) Physico Mechanical Process

- Spray drying and congealing
- Air suspension
- Solvent evaporation
- Pan coating

5.6.1 Chemical Methods

5.6.1.1 Interfacial Polymerization

This process involves in the dispersion of organic phase containing core material into the liquid manufacturing vehicle containing monomers, whereby the monomer reacts at the liquid/liquid interface to form a continuous layer. The capsule shell will be formed at the surface or on the surface of the droplet or particle by polymerization of the reactive monomers. A cross- linking agent may be added to the continuous phase to effect polymerization at interface. This method is suitable for low melting point solids or poorly soluble organic liquids

5.6.1.2 *In situ* Polymerization

In this process, no reactive agents are added to the core material. Polymerization occurs exclusively in the continuous phase and all polymerization occurs in the continuous phase, rather than on both sides of the interface between the continuous phase and the dispersed core material. Initially a low molecular weight pre polymer will be formed, as time goes on the pre polymer grows in size, and it deposits on the surface of the dispersed core material there by generating solid capsule shell. *E.g.* encapsulation of various water immiscible liquids with shells formed by the reaction at acidic pH of urea with formaldehyde in aqueous media.

5.6.2 Physico-chemical Methods

5.6.2.1 Coacervation and Phase Separation

This process consists of three steps:

(a) Formation of three immiscible chemical phases

(b) Deposition of the encapsulation

(c) Rigidization of the encapsulation

(a) Formation of three immiscible chemical phases

(i) Liquid manufacturing vehicle phase

(ii) Core material phase

(iii) Coating material phase.

Core material is dispersed in a solution of the polymer. The solvent for the polymer being the liquid manufacturing vehicle phase. The coating material phase, an immiscible polymer in a liquid state, is formed by utilizing one of the methods of phase separation or coacervation.

Methods for formation of three immiscible chemical phases:

(i) ***Temperature change*:** It involves the change in temperature, which results in separation of phases. With decrease in temperature, one phase become polymer poor (micro-encapsulation vehicle phase) and second phase (coating material phase) become polymer rich. Phase separation of the dissolved polymer occurs in the form of immiscible droplets.

Under proper polymer concentration, temperature, and agitation condition, liquid polymer droplets coalesce around the dispersed core material particle, this result in formation of embryonic microcapsule.

E.g.: Ethyl cellulose in cyclohexane (N-acetyl P-amino phenol as core)

(ii) ***Incompatible polymer addition*:** Liquid phase separation of a polymeric coating material and microencapsulation can be accomplished by utilizing the incompatibility of dissimilar polymer existing in a common solvent.

E.g.: Addition of polybutadiene to the solution of ethyl cellulose in toluene

(iii) ***Non solvent addition***: This method involves the addition of a liquid that is a non solvent for a given polymer to a solution of the polymer, to induce phase separation.

E.g.: Addition of isopropyl ether to methyl ethyl ketone solution of cellulose acetate butyrate

(iv) ***Salt addition***: It involves the addition of soluble inorganic salts to aqueous solution of certain water soluble polymers to cause phase separation.

E.g.: Addition of sodium sulphate solution to gelatin solution in vitamin encapsulation.

(v) ***Polymer-Polymer interaction***: It involves the interaction of oppositely charged polyelectrolyte, which results in formation of a complex having a reduced solubility that causes phase separation.

E.g.: Interaction of gum Arabic and gelatin at their iso-electric point.

(b) Deposition of the encapsulation

This process consists of depositing the liquid polymer coating upon the core material. This is accomplished by controlled physical mixing of the coating material and the core material in the manufacturing vehicle. Deposition of the liquid polymer coating around the core material occurs if the polymer is adsorbed at the interface formed between the core material and the liquid vehicle phase.

(c) Rigidization of the encapsulation

Rigidization is done by thermal, cross-linking or desolvation techniques to form self-sustaining microcapsules. Cross-linking is the formation of chemical links between molecular chains to form a three-dimensional network of connected molecules. The vulcanization of rubber using elemental sulphur is an example of cross-linking.

5.6.2.2 Polymer Encapsulation by Rapid Expansion of Supercritical Fluids

Supercritical fluids are highly compressed gasses that possess several advantageous properties of both liquids and gases. The most widely used being supercritical carbon dioxide (CO_2), alkanes (C_2 to C_4), and nitrous oxide (N_2O). A small change in temperature or pressure causes a large change in the density of supercritical fluids near the critical point. Supercritical CO_2 is widely used for its low critical temperature value, in addition to its nontoxic, non-flammable properties; it is also readily available, highly pure and cost-effective. The most widely used methods are as follows:

(a) Rapid expansion of supercritical solution (RESS)

(b) Gas anti-solvent (GAS) process

(c) Particles from gas-saturated solution (PGSS)

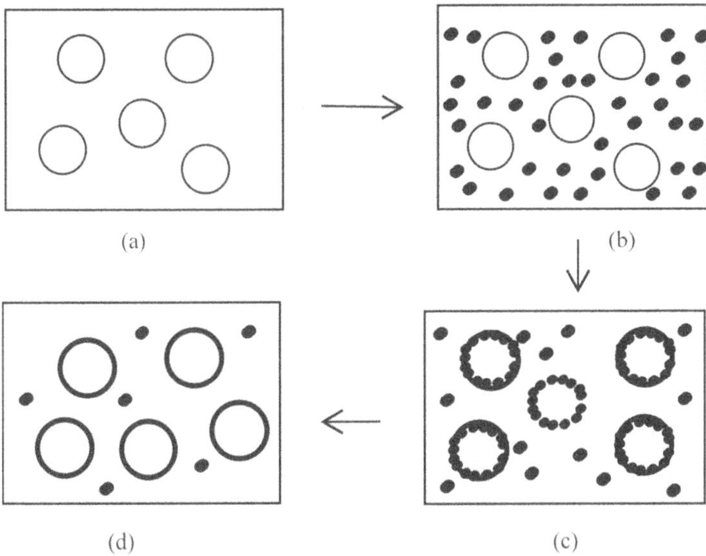

FIGURE 5.2 Schematic representation of the coacervation process. (a) Core material dispersion in solwution of shell polymer; (b) separation of coacervate from the solution; (c) coating of core material by micro droplets of coacervate; (d) coalescence of coacervate to form continuous shell around core particles.

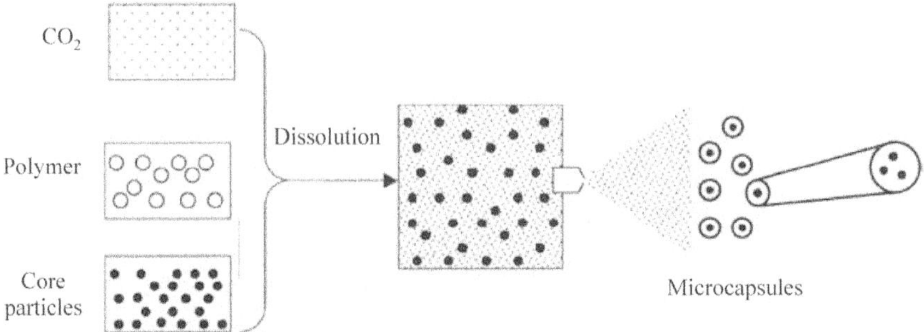

FIGURE 5.3 Microencapsulation by rapid expansion of supercritical solutions

(a) ***Rapid expansion of Supercritical Solution (RESS):*** In this process, supercritical fluid containing the active ingredient and the shell material are maintained at high pressure and then released at atmospheric pressure through a small nozzle. The sudden drop in pressure causes desolvation of the shell material, which is then deposited around the active ingredient (core) and forms a coating layer.

(b) ***Gas Anti-solvent (Gas) process:*** This process is also called supercritical fluid anti-solvent (SAS). In this method supercritical fluid is added to a solution of shell material and the active ingredients, and these are maintained at high pressure. This leads to a volume expansion of the solution that causes super saturation so that precipitation of the solute occurs.

(c) ***Particles from Gas-saturated Solution (PGSS):*** This process is carried out by mixing core and shell materials in supercritical fluid at high pressure. Swelling occurs during the process as supercritical fluid penetrates the shell material. When the mixture is heated above the glass transition temperature (Tg), the polymer undergoes liquefaction and the shell material deposits onto the active ingredient after releasing the pressure. In this process, the core and shell materials may not be soluble in the supercritical fluid.

5.6.3 Physico-mechanical Methods

5.6.3.1 Spray Drying and Spray Congealing

Spray drying is a mechanical microencapsulation method developed in the 1930s. Spray drying and spray congealing processes are similar, both involve the dispersion of core material in a liquefied coating substance and spraying or introducing the core- coating mixture into same environmental condition, whereby rapid solidification of the coating is affected by evaporation of solvent yielding the microcapsules, which are of polynuclear or matrix type. This process is applicable for both solids and liquids. The size of the microspheres obtained by this technology are ranging from 5 to 600 microns. Spray congealing can be done by spray drying equipment where coating will be applied as a melt. Core material is dispersed in a coating material melt rather than a coating solution. Coating solidification is accomplished by spraying the hot mixture into cool air stream or by dissolving in a non solvent. (*E.g.*: Waxes, fatty acids, and alcohols) Polymers which are solids at room temperature but meltable at reasonable temperature are applicable to spray congealing.

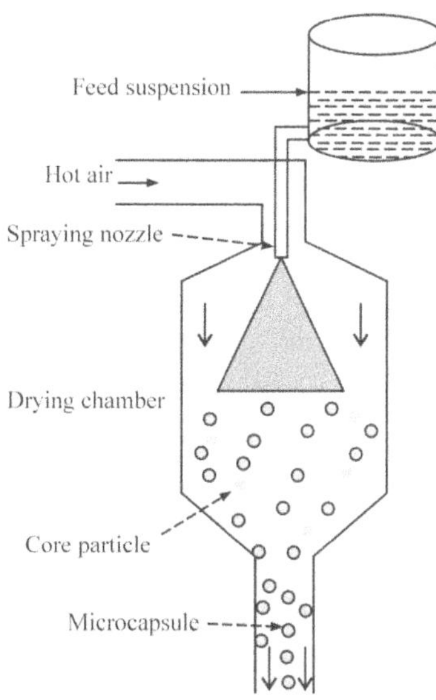

FIGURE 5.4 **Schematic illustrating the process of** micro-encapsulation by spray drying.

5.6.3.2 Air Suspension

This process consists of dispersing of solid, particulate core materials in a supporting air stream and spray coating of the air suspended particles is done. It is also known as Wurster process. The liquid coating is sprayed onto the particles and the rapid evaporation helps in the formation of an outer layer on the particles. The thickness and formulation of the coating can be obtained as desired. Different types of fluid-bed coaters include top spray, bottom spray, and tangential spray. This process is applicable only for the encapsulation of solid core material. Particle size ranges from 35-5000 microns.

(a) ***Top spray*:** In the top spray system the coating material is sprayed downwards on to the fluid bed so that as the solid or porous particles move to the coating region they become encapsulated.

(b) ***Bottle spray*:** The bottom spray technique uses a coating chamber that has a cylindrical nozzle and a perforated bottom plate. The cylindrical nozzle is used for spraying the coating material. As the particles move upwards through the perforated bottom plate and pass the nozzle area, the coating material encapsulates them.

(c) ***Tangential spray*:** The tangential spray consists of a rotating disc at the bottom of the coating chamber, with the same diameter as the chamber. During the process the disc is raised to create a gap between the edge of the chamber and the disc. The tangential nozzle is placed above the rotating disc through which the coating material is released. The particles move through the gap into the spraying zone and are encapsulated. As they travel a minimum distance there is a higher yield of encapsulated particles.

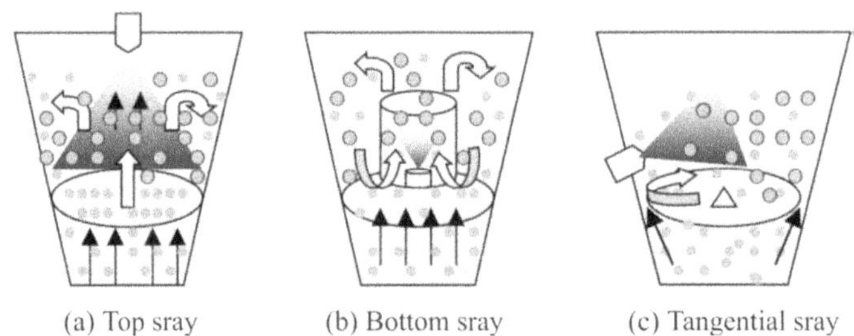

FIGURE 5.5 Schematics of a fluid-bed coater (a) Top spray; (b) bottom spray;(c) tangential spray.

5.6.3.3 Solvent Evaporation

This process is applicable for solids and liquids. The coating material is dissolved in a volatile solvent, which is immiscible with the liquid manufacturing vehicle phase. A core material to be encapsulated is dissolved or dispersed in the coating polymer solution. This mixture is added to the liquid manufacturing vehicle phase with agitation, the mixture is heated to evaporate the solvent for polymer. Here the coat material shrinks around the core material and encapsulate the core. Micro spheres of 5-fluorouracil have been prepared, using three grades of ethyl cellulose as wall forming materials, and utilizing a solvent evaporation technique under ambient conditions.

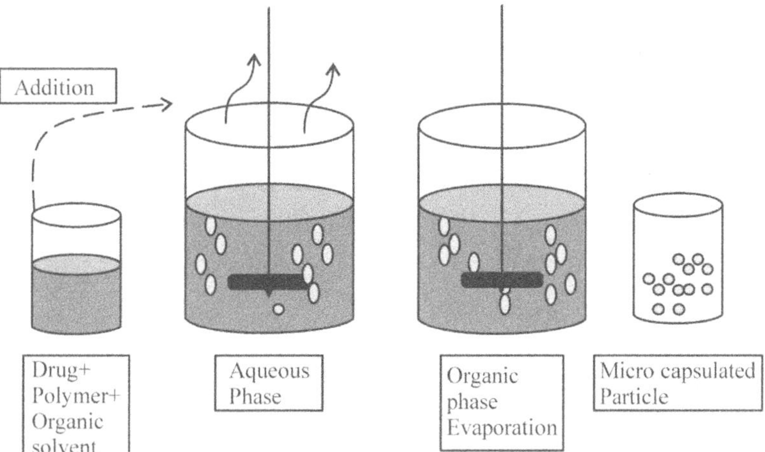

FIGURE 5.6 Solvent evaporation technique

5.6.3.4 Pan Coating

This process is suitable for micro encapsulation of large solid particles. Particle size ranges from 600- 5000 microns. The coating solution is applied as atomized spray to the solid core material in the coating pan. To remove the coating solvent warm air is passed over the coated material. By using this technique, larger sized particles will be coated effectively.

5.7   Mechanisms of Drug Release

Major mechanisms of drug release from microcapsules include diffusion, dissolution, osmosis and erosion

Diffusion: Diffusion is the most commonly involved mechanism wherein the dissolution fluid penetrates the shell, dissolves the core and leak out through the interstitial channels or pores. The kinetics of such drug release obey Higuchi's equation.

Dissolution: Dissolution rate of polymer coat determines the release rate of drug from the microcapsule when the coat is soluble in the dissolution fluid. Thickness of coat and its solubility in the dissolution fluid influence the release rate

Osmosis: The polymer coat of microcapsule acts as semi permeable membrane and allows the creation of an osmotic pressure difference between the inside and the outside of the microcapsule and drives drug solution out of the microcapsule through small pores in the coat.

Erosion: Erosion of coat due to pH and/or enzymatic hydrolysis causes drug release with certain coat materials like glyceryl monostearate, bee's wax and stearyl alcohol.

5.8   Evaluation

(a) *Drug entrapment efficiency*: The amount of drug present in the microcapsule is determined by extracting the drug into buffer under magnetic stirring for a period of approximately 2 hr. The solution is filtered through filter paper. Sample is suitably diluted and estimated for drug content spectrophotometrically.

(b) *Size distribution of microcapsules*: Size of microcapsules is determined by optical microscopy.

(c) *Shape and surface morphology*: The shape and surface morphology of the drug loaded microcapsules is investigated by using scanning electron microscope.

(d) *In-Vitro* **drug release study:** *In-vitro* drug release study is carried out in USP type I (Basket type) dissolution apparatus. Microcapsules are placed in the basket and immersed in the dissolution medium maintained at 37 ± 5 °c and stirred for specified period. Samples are withdrawn at different time intervals; Withdrawn samples are analysed spectrophotometrically.

5.9 Recent Advancement in Microencapsulation

The preparation of polymeric micro particles recently gained a vide importance in the field of microencapsulation. The term micro particle designates systems larger than one micrometer in diameter and is used usually to describe both microcapsules and microspheres. The purpose behind the formulation of micro particles containing drugs are employed for controlling the release of drug, masking the taste and odour of drugs, protection of the drugs from degradation, and protection of the body from the toxic effects of the drugs. An erodible or a non-erodible type of polymeric carriers are used in micro particle fabrication.

Microspheres and microcapsules are established as unique carrier systems for many pharmaceuticals and can be tailored to adhere to targeted tissue systems.

- A micro particle carrier based system of several drugs (Minocycline HCl) prepared using biodegradable polymer has been used to deliver drug to a posterior part of an eye of a mammal to treat or prevent a disease or condition affecting mammals.

- A method has been developed for preparing enteric coated polymer micro particles containing a proteinaceous antigen in a single or double emulsification process in which the enteric polymer acts as a stabilizer for the micro particles which are formed in the process.

- **Microencapsulation of bioactive substances:** A new, innovative and natural encapsulant material allows targeted delivery of susceptible or unpalatable ingredients such as omega-3.

- **Microencapsulation of probiotics for industrial applications and targeted delivery:**
  Probiotics are live microbial feed supplements that beneficially affect the host by improving its intestinal microbial balance.

- **Encapsulation of nucleotides and growth hormone using simple or double emulsification methods.**

- **Oral delivery of Insulin by using various microencapsulation techniques:** Main aim is protecting insulin from enzymatic degradation in stomach.

- **Microencapsulation in treatment of endodontic and periodontal diseases:** The controlled release from polymer micro particles enables therapeutic levels of drugs to be reached in periodontal or dental treatments by modifying the physicochemical properties of microspheres or the appropriate selection of materials for the formulation.

- **Encapsulating DNA:** A novel method of encapsulating DNA, help sretaining its ability to induce expression of its coding sequence in a micro particle for oral administration prepared using the w/o/w emulsion and using biodegradable polymers.

6 Liquid Dosage Forms

Introduction

Liquid dosage forms such as, solutions, suspensions, and emulsions offer unique advantages when compared to conventional tablets and capsules, from ease in dosing to ease in administration. One of the most desirable features of liquid dosage formulation is that it has relatively effective bioavailability as there is no dissolution time and rapid absorption from the stomach/intestines is possible when compared to tablets. Apart from the various advantages, a number of challenges occur related to the formulation and development of these liquid dosage forms. These include stability problems, need for taste masking, phase separations and all these dosage forms require highly specialized formulation techniques.

6.1 Solutions

Solutions are one of the oldest dosage forms used in the treatment of patients and offer rapid and high absorption of soluble medicinal products. Therefore, the compounding of solutions retains an important place in therapeutics today. Owing to the simplicity and the speed of preparation of an ad hoc formulation, they are of particular use for individuals who have difficulty in swallowing solid dosage forms (for example paediatric, geriatric, intensive care and psychiatric patients), where compliance needs to be checked on administration (for example in prisons or psychiatric pharmacy) and in cases where precise, individualized dosages are required.

Solution is a homogeneous liquid preparation that contains one or more dissolved active ingredients with or without excipients. Solutions are one of the oldest and most popular dosage forms owing to the simplicity and the speed of preparation.

The advantages and disadvantages of solutions are as follows:

Advantages

1. The drug is immediately available for absorption. By providing the drug in a solution, the dissolution phase of the absorption process can be bypassed, providing rapid absorption.

2. Flexible dosing is possible. The active ingredient within the solution will be present in a certain concentration per unit volume. If alterations to the quantity of active ingredient to be administered are required, a simple alteration to the quantity of solution to be taken is all that is required.

3. They may be designed for any route of absorption. Suitable for administering by various routes such as, oral, nasal, otic, ophthalmic, paternterals etc).

4. Easy for swallowing, particularly for individuals who have difficulty in swallowing solid dosage forms (for example paediatric, geriatric, intensive care and psychiatric patients).

Disadvantages

1. Drug stability is often reduced in solution by solvolysis, hydrolysis or oxidation.

2. It is difficult to mask unpleasant tastes.

3. They are bulky, difficult to transport and prone to breakage there by loss of the preparation occurs.

4. Accurate dose precision is not there as patients abilities to measure an accurate dose can vary considerably.

5. Some drugs are poorly soluble. The solubility of a drug needs to be taken into consideration when preparing a solution to ensure that the final volume produced is not excessive.

6.1.1 Formulation Consideration

6.1.1.1 Excipients

Characteristics of active drug are of major concern in developing an oral liquid dosage formulation. The major challenges in developing oral liquid dosage forms are

- Stability of a drug in solution,
- Solubility of a drug at the required level,
- Acceptable taste.

By effective use of excipients, one can overcome these challenges. Excipients in pharmaceutical formulations are physiologically inert compounds that are included in the formulation to facilitate the proper administration of the dosage form, *e.g.*: pourability, palatability, protection, stability and to enhance the solubility of the therapeutic agent. Pharmaceutical solutions commonly contain a wide range of excipients, the details of which are provided below.

The excipients commonly required for any liquid formulation are vehicles (water/oil), viscosity modifiers, stabilizers, preservatives, antioxidants, colouring agents, sweeteners and flavours. In addition, solubilizers are required in case of solutions, suspending agents for suspensions and emulsifying agents for emulsions.

Vehicles: Vehicles are the liquid agents that carry drugs and other excipients in dissolved or dispersed state. Pharmaceutical vehicles can be classified as aqueous vehicles, such as water, hydro-alcoholic vehicles and oily vehicles such as, vegetable oils, mineral oils or emulsified bases.

Purified Water: Water is preferred as vehicle, as it is nontoxic, non-irritant, tasteless, relatively cheap, and many drugs are water soluble. Problems may be encountered where active drugs are not particularly water soluble or suffer from hydrolysis in aqueous solution. Ordinary drinking water is not acceptable for the manufacturing of most of the pharmaceutical preparations since it contains dissolved salts and incompatibility may occur with medicinal agents. Purified water united State pharmacopoeia is allowed for usage as vehicle or as a component of vehicle for aqueous liquid formulations. Purified water united state pharmacopoeia is prepared by distillation, reverse osmosis, ion exchange resin treatment, ozonization etc.

Efforts should be made to provide as much microbial-free water as possible; this can be readily achieved by installing a loop system in which the incoming water is first subjected to ultraviolet sterilizer, carbon filter, demineralizer, and a 5-micron filter, and then sent to a heated tank, from which it is passed again through an ultraviolet sterilizer and then a 0.22-micron filter before bringing it into the product; water coming out of the 5-micron filter can be circulated.

Non Aqueous vehicles

(a) Alcohol

(b) Polyhydric alcohol

- Glycerol glycerine
- Propylene glycol

(c) Fixed Oils

(a) *Alcohol***:** It is used at low concentrations as a cosolvent and exhibit antibacterial activity

(b) *Polyhydric alcohol***:** These are characterized by their lower volatility than monohydric alcohols. Examples of polyhydric alcohols are glycerol and Propylene glycol.

- *Glycerol (***Glycerine***)***:** It is a clear, colourless liquid, with thick, syrupy consistency, odourless, very sweet and slightly warm to the taste. Glycerin is used as vehicle in various pharmaceutical products. It is also used to improve viscosity, taste and flavour.

- *Propylene Glycol USP***:** Propylene glycol is an outstanding solvent for many organic compounds. It is colourless, odourless and has a very slight characteristic taste. The toxicity of propylene glycol is quite less in comparison to many other cosolvents generally used.

(c) *Fixed oils***:** Used for the formulation of emulsions.

Sweetening Agents: Taste is of prime importance in the administration of liquid products. Sweetening agents are employed in liquid formulations designed for oral administration specifically to increase the palatability of the therapeutic agent. Often a combination of sweetening agents is used, in combination with various flavours (which are often included to make the product more palatable), to impart the best taste.

Natural sweetening agents are low molecular weight carbohydrate such as sucrose and polyhydric alcohols such as sorbitol, mannitol, fructose and liquid sugar.

Artificial sweetening agents (Intense sweeteners) are sodium saccharine, Aspartame Ocesulfame and Thaumatin.

- *Sodium/Calcium Saccharine***:** It is approximately 250-500 times sweeter than sugar. It has a high water solubility and physical and chemical stability over a wide range of pH. It is found to have bitter and metallic after taste and carcinogenic in nature.

- *Aspartame***:** It is the methyl ester of aspartic acid and phenyl alanine. It is approximately 200 times sweeter than sugar. It has no bitter after taste. Its stability in aqueous solution is pH dependent.

Flavouring Agents: These are used to make disagreeable taste of the product more palatable. Flavour is a complex blend of taste and odour. There are four basic sensations: salty, bitter, sweet, and sour. A combination of efforts is required to mask these tastes. A large number of natural and artificial flavours and their combinations are available to mask the bitterness most often. Menthol and chloroform act as desensitizing agents. The colour of the product must have psychogenic balance with taste and odour as depicted in Table 6.1.

TABLE 6.1

Taste and flavour selection

Taste	Preferable flavour	Colour
Salty	Peach, Apricot	Yellow, white, green
Bitter	Chocolate, mint, Wild cherry	Brown, Red
Sweet	Vanilla, Rose	White, pink,
Sour	Citrus fruits, Raspberry	Yellow, green, orange

In some cases, there exists a strong association between the use of a product and its flavours for example; for indigestion mint; for cough cherry and mint for antacid lemon, fruity.

Colouring Agents: A colourant is an integral part of liquid oral formulation to improve elegance. Colour of liquid products is often synchronized with the flavours used; for example, brown or red for chocolate, white for vanilla, and so forth. Various FD & C certified natural and artificial colours in the form of dyes, pigments and lakes are used.

Viscosity Modifiers: An appropriate control of viscosity is required to allow good dosing control as the flow of liquid for dispensing and dosing is important. Many thickening agents are available including carboxymethyl cellulose, methyl cellulose, polyvinyl pyrrolidone, and sugar.

Preservatives: Preservatives are almost always a part of liquid formulations and act by various mechanism such as, modification of cell membrane, coagulation of proteins, cytoplasmic lysis, oxidation of cellular components and hydrolysis.

Ideal qualities of preservatives are as follows:

- Should be effective in minimum concentration
- Should be effective over a wide range of microorganism
- Should not affect safety of the patient i.e., should be non-sensitizing and non-irritating

- Should have adequate stability during shelf life
- Should be compatible with the other excipients
- Should not affect container or the product

Classifications of preservatives are as follows:

Preservatives can be classified as acidic, neutral, mercurial and quaternary as shown in table 6.2 and their minimum effective ranges are shown in Table 6.3.

TABLE 6.2

Classifications of preservatives

Class of Preservatives	Examples
Acidic	Phenol, chlorocresol, o-pheyl phenol, alkyl esters of parahydroxybenzoic acid, benzoic acid and its salts, boric acid and its salts, and sorbic acid and its salts;
Neutral	Chlorbutanol, Benzyl alcohol, and beta-phenylethyl alcohol;
Mercurial	Thiomersal, Phenylmercuric acetate, and nitrate; and Nitromersol;
Quarternary compounds	Benzalkonium chloride and cetylpyridinium chloride.

TABLE 6.3

Concentration range for preservatives

Name of preservatives	Concentration range%
Disodiumedentate	0.1
Benzalkonium chloride	0.01-0.02
Benzoicacid	0.1
Butylparaben	0.006-0.05
Cetrimide	0.005
Chlorobutanol	0.5
Phenylmercuric acetate	0.001-0.002
Sodiumbenzoate	0.02-0.5
Methylparaben	0.015-0.2

Antioxidants: Antioxidants are the agents which inhibit oxidation. Antioxidants undergo oxidation in place of drug or they block the oxidation reaction or they act as synergists to other antioxidants.

Chelators may also act as antioxidant. Examples of antioxidants that are commonly used for aqueous formulations include: sodium sulphite, sodium metabisulphite, sodium formaldehyde sulphoxylate and ascorbic acid. Examples of antioxidants that may be used in oil-basedsolutions include: butylated hydroxytoluene (BHT), butylatedhydroxyanisole (BHA) and propyl gallate.

TABLE 6.4

Classification of antioxidants

Antioxidants	Examples
Chelating agents	Citric acid, EDTA, Typtophane, tartaric acid
Preferentially oxidized	Ascorbic acid, Sodium sulphite, sodium bi sulphite
Chain terminator	CysteineHC, Thioglycolic acid,
Water Soluble	Thiosorbitol, thioglycerol
Water Insoluble	Alkyl gallte, BHT, BHA, α-tocopherol

pH Modifiers: To prevent large changes in liquid formulation during storage control of the pH is important. Buffers are used in the liquid products to modify the solubility of drugs and drug stability.

Examples of buffer salts used in pharmaceutical solutions include:

- Acetates (acetic acid and sodium acetate): 1-2%
- Citrates (citric acid and sodium citrate): 1-5%
- Phosphates (sodium phosphate and disodium phosphate): 0.8-2%.

Wetting Agents/Solubility Enhancer: Wetting agents are used in liquid dosage forms to create a homogenous dispersion of solid particlesin a liquid vehicle. Wetting agents are surfactants having HLB (hydrophile-lipophile balance) value 7-9 lowers the contact angle and aid in spread ability of water on the particles surface to displace the air layer at the surface and help in wetting and solubilisation.

The most common solubilizers used include polyoxyethylene sorbital, fatty acid esters, polyoxyethylene monoalklyl ethers, sucrose monoesters, lanolin esters and ether.

Different Types of Liquid Dosage Form

- *Syrups*: A syrup is a concentrated, viscous solution containing one or more sugar components, chiefly sucrose.

- ***Mixtures***: Simple liquid preparations intended for oral use containing dissolved medicaments may be described as oral solutions or mixtures, although the term 'mixture' may also be applied to a suspension.

- ***Draughts***: It is a term used to describe a single dose liquid preparation, which is larger than generally used volume in traditional mixture formulations. Each draught is usually supplied in a 50 mL unit dose container.

- ***Linctus***: A linctus is a liquid oral preparation that is chiefly used for a demulcent, expectorant or sedative purpose, principally in the treatment of cough.

- ***Elixirs***: An elixir is a clear, hydro alcoholic liquid preparation containing a high proportion of sugar or other sweetening agent, included to mask offensive or nauseating tastes.

- ***Spirits***: Spirits are solutions containing one or more active medicaments dissolved in either absolute or dilute ethanol.

- ***Gargles and mouthwashes***: Gargles and mouth washes are aqueous solutions that are intended for treatment of the throat (gargles) and mouth (mouthwashes) and are generally formulated in a concentrated form. These preparations must be diluted before use and are not intended to be swallowed.

- ***Paediatric drops***: These are oral liquid formulation of medicament usually in solution, intended for administration to paediatrics. The formulation is designed to have very small dose volumes which must be administered with a calibrated dropper.

Disperse systems: The term disperse system refers to a system in which one of the phase (the dispersed phase) is distributed, in discrete units, throughout a second phase (the continuous phase). Classification of dispersed systems on the basis of particle size is shown in Table 6.5.

TABLE 6.5

Types of dispersed systems

	Type	Size	Examples
1	Molecular dispersion	< 1 nm	Oxygen molecules, glucose solution
2	Colloidal dispersion	1nm- 0.5 mm	1. Natu 2. ral polymers
3	Coarse dispersion	> 0.5 mm	Suspension and emulsion

6.2 Suspension

A pharmaceutical suspension can be defined as a thermodynamically unstable coarse dispersed system containing finely divided insoluble material suspended in a liquid medium which is stabilized with the help of suspending agents. Generally pharmaceutical suspensions contain aqueous dispersion phase however in some cases they may be an oily or organic phase. The suspensions have dispersed particles above the colloidal size, i.e., mean particle diameter above 1 µm.

Suspensions are manufactured either by a precipitation or by dispersed methods requiring use of suspending agents whose characteristics can significantly change because of the presence of other components such as electrolytes.

Ideal Properties of Suspensions:

- Suspensions should possess sufficient viscosity and good pour ability leading to ease of removal of dose from container.
- The particle should not form a cake on settling.
- The dispersed particles should not settle readily and if settled should be redispersed immediately on shacking.
- They should have good organoleptic properties.
- It should be palatable.
- The particle size distribution should be uniform.
- They should be physically and chemically stable.
- They should be resistant against microbial contamination.

Advantages

- Suspension can improve chemical stability of certain drug. *E.g.*: Procaine penicillin G.
- Drug in suspension exhibits higher rate of bioavailability than other dosage forms.
- Duration and onset of action can be controlled. *E.g.*: Protamine zinc-Insulin suspension.
- Suspension can mask the unpleasant/bitter taste of drug. *E.g.* Chloramphenicol.
- Suspension is usually applicable for drugs which are insoluble or poorly soluble. *E.g.*: Prednisolone suspension.

Disadvantages

- Physical stability, sedimentation and compaction can cause problems.
- It is bulky hence sufficient care must be taken during handling and transport.
- It is difficult to formulate.
- Uniform and accurate dose cannot be achieved unless suspension are packed in unit dosage form.

6.2.1 Types of Suspensions

Suspensions are classified as:

1. **Based on Size of Solid Particles**
   - Colloidal suspension (1 nm to 0.5 μm)
   - Coarse suspension (1 to 100 μm)
   - Nano suspension (10 nm)

2. **According to the Route of Administration**
   - Oral suspensions should be taken by oral route
   - Topical suspensions meant for external application
   - Parenteral suspensions should be sterile and should possess property of syring ability.
   - Ophthalmic suspensions should be sterile and should be made of very fine particles.

3. **According to the Nature of Dispersed Phase and Methods of Preparation**

   These suspensions are classified as suspensions containing diffusible solids, indiffusible solids, poorly wettable solids, precipitate forming liquids and products of chemical reactions.

4. **Based on Electro Kinetic Nature of Solid Particles**

   *Flocculated Suspensions***:** In this system solid particles of dispersed phase aggregates to form loose network like structure of solid particles in dispersion medium. The aggregates form no hard cake. These aggregates settle rapidly due to their size as rate of sedimentation is high and sediment formed is loose and easily re-dispersible. The suspension is not elegant; as dispersed phase tends to separate out from the dispersion medium.

***Deflocculated Suspensions*:** In this types of suspensions the solid particles exist as separate entities in dispersion medium. The sediments form hard cake. The solid drug particles settle slowly as rate of sedimentation is low. As sediments are formed eventually there is difficulty of redispersion. The suspension is more elegant as dispersed phase remain suspended for a long time giving uniform appearance.

TABLE 6.6

Difference between flocculated and deflocculated suspension

Flocculated	Deflocculated
1. Particles forms loose aggregates	3. Particles exist as separate discreet unit
2. Rate of sedimentation is high	4. Rate of sedimentation is slow
3. Sediment is loosely packed and does not form a hard cake	5. Sediment is very closely packed and a hard cake is formed
4. Sediment is easy to redisperse	6. Sediment is difficult to redisperse
5. The floccules stick to the sides of the bottle	7. They don't stick to the sides of the bottle

5. Based on Proportion of Solid Particles

- Dilute suspension (2 to10%w/v solid)
- Concentrated suspension (50%w/v solid)

6.2.2 Formulation of Suspension

The various additives, which are used in suspension formulation, are as follows.

TABLE 6.7

Components and their functions

Additives	Function
Wetting agents	To disperse solids in continuous liquid phase.
Suspending/Flocculating agents	To suspend the drug particles
Thickeners	To increase the viscosity of suspension.
Buffers/pH adjusting agents	To stabilize the suspension to a desired pH range.
Colouring agents	To impart desired colour to suspension and improve elegance.
Preservatives	To prevent microbial growth.
Structured liquid vehicle	To construct structure of the final suspension.

Suspending Agents/Thickening Agents

Suspending agents also act as thickening agents. They are added with the objective to increase apparent viscosity of the continuous phase thus preventing rapid sedimentation of the dispersed particles. which is necessary to prevent sedimentation of the suspended particles as per Stroke's law. Most suspending agents perform two functions i.e., besides acting as a suspending agent they also impart viscosity to the solution. Suspending agents form film around particle and decrease interparticular attraction. A good suspension should have well developed thixotropy. At rest the solution should be sufficiently viscous to prevent sedimentation and thus aggregation or caking of the particles. When agitation is applied the viscosity is reduced and provide good flow characteristic from the mouth of bottle. Use of combination of suspending agents may give beneficial action as compared to single suspending agent. Some important characteristics of most commonly used suspending agents are:

A. Natural Polysaccharides

Acacia: It is the dry exudate obtained from stems and branches of various species of Acacia. It has low thickening properties but it is a good protective colloid. It is used in combination with tragacanth and starch for internal preparations. Acacia mucilage becomes acidic on storage as a result of enzymatic activity.

Tragacanth: Gum Tragacanth is dried exudate obtained from Astragalus gummifer or another species of Astragalus. It is widely used as suspending agent. Tragacanth forms viscous solution or gels with water and most stable at pH values between 4 and 7.5. Tragacanth is non-toxic and almost tasteless and is widely used in suspensions for internal use.

Sodium Alginate: Sodium Alginate consists of purified carbohydrate product extracted from brown seaweeds by use of dilute alkali. It chiefly consists of sodium salt of alginic acid. Various grades are usually available commercially for different applications and yield solutions of various viscosities. Sodium Alginate is slowly soluble in water. Alginate solution loses its viscosity when heated above 60 °C due to depolymerization. Fresh solution has highest viscosity, after which viscosity gradually decreases and acquires constant value after 24 hrs. Maximum viscosity is observed at a pH range of 5-9.

***Xanthan Gum*:** Xanthan Gum consists of the purified polysaccharide gum obtained by fermentation of a carbohydrate by bacteria of genus *Xanthomonas* chiefly *Xanthomonas campestris*. It is soluble in hot and cold water and produces a viscous product that is stable over a wide range of temperature and pH in comparison to tragacanth, it is easier to use and is capable of preparing suspensions of better quality and improved consistency.

B. Semi-Synthetic Polysaccharides

***Methyl Cellulose*:** It consists of the ethyl ether derivative of cellulose. It is dispersed slowly in cold water to form colloidal solution but is insoluble in hot water. Methyl cellulose is non-ionic and is stable over a wide range of pH values. Methylcellulose is available in several viscosity grades depending upon the degree of methylation and polymer chain length. On heating to 50 °C, solution of methylcellulose is converted to gel form and on cooling, it is again converted to solution form. Methylcellulose is not susceptible to microbial growth and is non-toxic.

***Hydroxyethyl Cellulose*:** It consists of the hydroxyl ethyl ether derivative of cellulose and is mainly used as viscosity increasing agent. Unlike methyl cellulose. It is soluble in cold as well as hot water and produces a clear solution that is stable even at higher temperatures. Various grades are available that differ in their aqueous viscosities. Solution display maximum stability in pH range 2 to 10.

***Sodium Carboxymethyl Cellulose (Na-CMC)*:** It is also known as Carmellose Sodium; it consists of the sodium salt of Carboxy methyl ether derivative of cellulose. Different viscosity grades are available. It is soluble in hot as well as cold water forming stable mucilage within the range of 5 and 10. Being anionic, it is incompatible with the cationic compounds. Available in low, medium and high viscosity grades.

***Microcrystalline Cellulose (MCC)*:** It is not soluble in water, but it readily disperses in water to give thixotropic gels. It is used in combination with Na-CMC, MC or HPMC, because they facilitate dispersion of MCC.

***Hydroxypropyl Methyl Cellulose (HPMC)*:** It is also known as Hypermellose; it consists of the hydroxypropyl derivative of methyl cellulose. It has properties similar to those of methyl cellulose but produces aqueous solutions with higher gelling points. Various grades are available that differ in their aqueous solution viscosities.

C. Synthetic Agents

Carbomer: Carbomer is a high molecular weight polymer of acrylic acid cross linked with alkyl sucrose. It disperses in water to form an acidic colloidal solution of low viscosity. Several viscosity grades are available and the concentration used varies from 0.1% to 4% as suspending agent. Carbomer gels are most viscous between pH 6 and 11. The viscosity is reduced on lowering the pH to below 3 or rising above 12. Carbomer is susceptible to oxidation especially on exposure to light and hence formulations should be stabilized by addition of appropriate antioxidants and chelating agents.

Colloidal Silicon dioxide: This is a form of Silicon dioxide having colloidal dimensions. It acts as a suspending agent by forming aggregates which associates to form three dimensional networks, thus preventing sedimentation in a concentration between 1.5 to 4%.

D. Clays

Clays are inorganic materials, mainly hydrated silicates derived from natural sources. They form highly thixotropic gels.

Aluminium Magnesium Silicate: Also known as Veegum, Aluminium Magnesium Silicate is mainly used at a concentration range of 0.5% to 2% as a suspending agent for both internal and external preparations. A number of different grades are available; which are distinguished by the degree of alkalinity and the viscosity of an aqueous dispersion. Dispersions in water are thixotropic, and at a concentration of 10% a firm gel is obtained.

Bentonite: Bentonite is a natural colloidal hydrated aluminium silicate when it gets. In contact with water it forms either sols or gels depending on its concentration. It is generally used at a concentration range between 0.5% to 2% and shows maximum stability at pH values between 3 and 10.

Hectorite: Hectorite is a natural colloidal magnesium silicate having properties similar to bentonite. It swells up to 36 times its original volume and forms highly thixotropic gels at concentration of 1 to 2%.

TABLE 6.8

Types of suspending agents

Suspending agents	Stability pH range	Conc. used
Sodium alginate	4-10	1– 5 %
Methyl cellulose	3-11	1– 2 %
Hydroxy ethyl cellulose	2-12	1-2%
Hydroxypropyl cellulose	6-8	1-2%
Hydroxy propyl methyl cellulose	3-11	1-2%
CMC	7-9	1-2%
Na-CMC	5-10	0.1-5%
Micro crystalline cellulose	1-11	0.6– 1.5 %
Tragacanth	4-8	1-5%
Xanthangum	3-12	0.05-0.5%
Bentonite	> 6	0.5– 5.0 %
Carrageenan	6-10	0.5– 1 %
Guargum	4-10.5	1-5%
Colloidal silicon dioxide	0-7.5	2– 4 %

Wetting Agents: Wetting agents are additives which are usually added to reduce hydrophobicity. These agents generally get adsorbed at the solid-liquid interface and promote wetting of the solid particles by the liquid of the dispersion medium. A variety of substances including have been employed as wetting agents. Non-ionic surfactants are most commonly used as wetting agents in pharmaceutical suspensions. Non-ionic surfactants having HLB value between 7-10 are best as wetting agents.

Surfactants: Surfactants act by decreasing the interfacial tension between drug particles and liquid and thus liquid is penetrated in the pores of drug particle displacing air from them. Generally, surfactants possessing HLB values between 7 and 9 have been employed as wetting agents. These orient themselves at solid-liquid interface and decrease the interfacial tension between the particles of the dispersed phase and the dispersed medium. Most surfactants are used at concentration of 0.1 to 0.2%. Examples of surfactants employed for oral preparation includes polysorbates, sorbitan, esters, etc., for external preparations, sodium lauryl sulfate, sodium dioctyl sulfosuccinate and quillia extracts can also be used.

Polysorbate 80 is most widely used due to its following advantages:

Advantages

- It is non-ionic so no change in pH of medium
- No toxicity. Safe for internal use.
- Less foaming tendencies, however it should be used at concentration less than 0.5%.
- Compatible with most of the adjuvant

Disadvantages

- It is adsorbed on plastic container decreasing its preservative action
- It interacts with preservatives such as methyl paraben and reduces antimicrobial activity.

Hydrophilic Colloids: Hydrophilic colloids act by coating the surface of hydrophobic particles and imparting hydrophilic character and facilitate wetting. Various hydrophilic colloids such as acacia, bentonite, colloidal silicon dioxide and cellulose derivatives have also been employed as wetting agents. These polymers have a linear branched chain structure and form a gel like network within the system. They get adsorbed on to the surface of the dispersed particles and hold them in a flocculated state.

Flocculating Agents: These are substances added to cause controlled aggregation of the particles of the dispersed phase in a suspension. Examples of such agents include surfactants, electrolytes and hydrophilic polymers.

Electrolytes: These acts by neutralizing the surface charge on the particles of the dispersed phase thereby reducing the electrical barrier between them. Electrolytes such as sodium salt of acetates, phosphates and citrates have been commonly employed as flocculating agents. The effectiveness of the electrolytes as flocculating agents depends on the valance of the ions of these electrolytes. Thus, divalent ions are ten times more effective than the monovalent ions while trivalent ones are thousand times more effective.

Structured Vehicles: Structured vehicles are pseudo plastic and plastic in nature. These act by entrapping the deflocculated particles so that no settling occurs and particles remain deflocculated and applying the principles of flocculation to produce floccules that settle rapidly with ease of dispersibility with a minimum agitation. The shear-thinning property of these vehicles facilitates the reformation of a uniform dispersion when shear is applied. Thus the product must flow readily from the container and possess a uniform distribution of particles in each dose.

6.2.3 Formulation of Suspensions

6.2.3.1 Dispersion Technique

Vehicle must be formulated so that the solid phase is easily wetted and dispersed. The use of surfactant is desirable to ensure uniform wetting of hydrophobic solids. The preparation of suspension includes three methods: (1) use of controlled flocculation and (2) use of structured vehicle (3) combination of both of the two pervious methods. The general guidelines to suspension formulation is as shown in Figure 6.1.

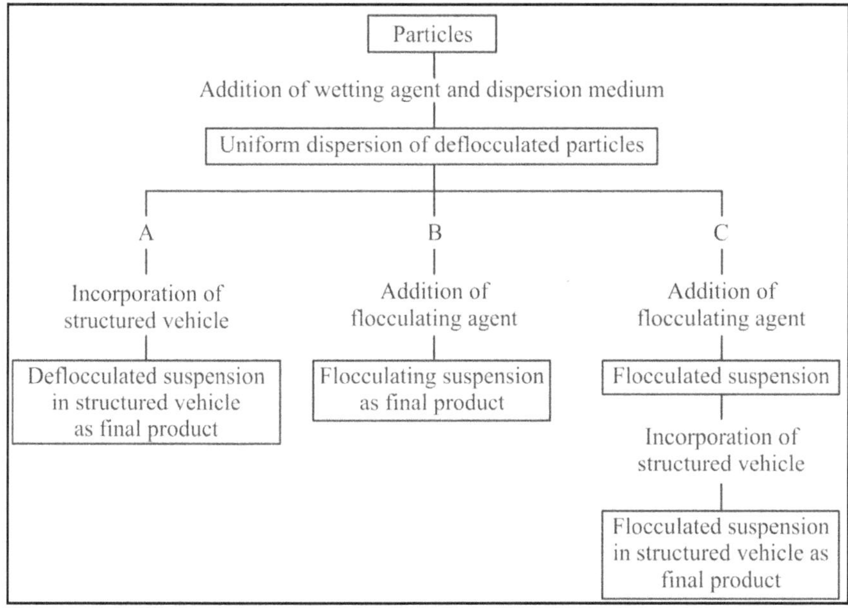

FIGURE 6.1 General guidelines for suspension formulation.

Suspensions containing diffusible solids consist of solids insoluble in water but easily wettable. On shaking with water solid particles diffuse readily throughout the liquid and remain suspended for a long time. The suspensions containing diffusible solids are prepared by triturating the solids in a mortar with sufficient quantity of vehicle to form a smooth cream. Any soluble nonvolatile substance is then added by separately dissolving them in a small quantity of vehicle. More vehicles and volatile component are added at this stage and adding the required quantity of vehicle makes up the final volume.

Example: Magnesium Trisilicate Mixture.

Suspensions containing indiffusible solids consist of substances, which do not remain distributed in the dispersion medium when shaken for long time to ensure uniformity of dose. They are prepared by adding a suitable thickening agent to the vehicle, which increases the viscosity of the vehicle and delays the separation or sedimentation of indiffusible particles.

Example: Calamine Lotion.

Suspensions containing poorly wettable solids consist of substances, which are poorly soluble, and at the same time poorly wetted by the dispersion medium, and clump together with the difficulty to disperse. They are prepared by including suitable wetting agent in the formulation. These agents get adsorbed at the solid/liquid interface and promote wetting of the solid particles by the liquid of the dispersion medium.

Example: Sulphur Lotion.

6.2.3.2 Precipitation Techniques

- Organic solvent precipitation.
- Precipitation effected by changing pH of medium-protaminezinc insulin.
- Double decomposition: Preparation of white lotion, that is forming zinc polysulphide by mixing zinc sulfate and sulfurated potash solutions.

Suspensions of precipitate forming liquids consist of liquid tinctures which are alcoholic or hydroalcoholic extract of vegetable drugs which contain resinous material. When tinctures are added to water they precipitate. Precipitates are indiffusible and stick to the walls of the container. They are prepared by adding a suitable thickening agent prior to the addition of the precipitate forming liquid.

Example: Lobelia and Stramonium Mixture.

6.2.3.3 Suspensions Produced by Chemical Reactions

These are prepared by mixing two dilute solutions of reactants to form a fine precipitate. Generally, precipitates so formed are diffusible and no suspending agent is required. If precipitate is indiffusible a suitable thickening or suspending agent may be added. They are prepared by dissolving the reactants separately in approximately half volumes of the vehicle and the two portions are then mixed together.

Example: Zinc Sulphide Lotion

6.2.4 Stability of Suspensions

The physical stability of a pharmaceutical suspension is the condition in which the particles do not aggregate and in which they remain uniformly distributed throughout the dispersions. Factors to be considered for the stability of suspension are:

6.2.4.1 Particle Size

Particle size of any suspension is critical and must be reduced within the range as determined during the preformulation study. Too large or too small particles should be avoided. Larger particles will settle faster at the bottom of the container and too fine particles will easily form hard cake at the bottom of the container.

6.2.4.2 Sedimentation

Sedimentation of particles in a suspension is governed by several factors: particle size, density of the particles, density of the vehicle, and viscosity of the vehicle. The velocity of sedimentation of particles in a suspension can be determined by using the Stokes's law:

$$V = \frac{d^2 g (\rho_p - \rho_s)}{18 \eta}$$

where

V = velocity of sedimentation

d = diameter of the particle

g = acceleration of gravity

ρ_1 = density of the particle

ρ_2 = density of the vehicle

η = viscosity of the vehicle

According to the Stoke's equation, the velocity of sedimentation of particles in a suspension can be reduced by decreasing the particle size and also by minimizing the difference between the densities of the particles and the vehicle.

6.2.4.3 Electro Kinetic Properties

Dispersed solid particles in a suspension may have charge in relation to their surrounding vehicle. These solid particles may become charged through one of two situations.

1. Selective adsorption of a particular ionic species is present in the vehicle. This may be due to the addition of some ionic species in a polar solvent. Consider a solid particle in contact with an electrolyte solution. The particle may become positively or negatively charged by selective adsorption of either cations or anions from the solution.

2. Ionization of functional group of the particle. In this situation, the total charge is a function of the pH of the surrounding vehicle.

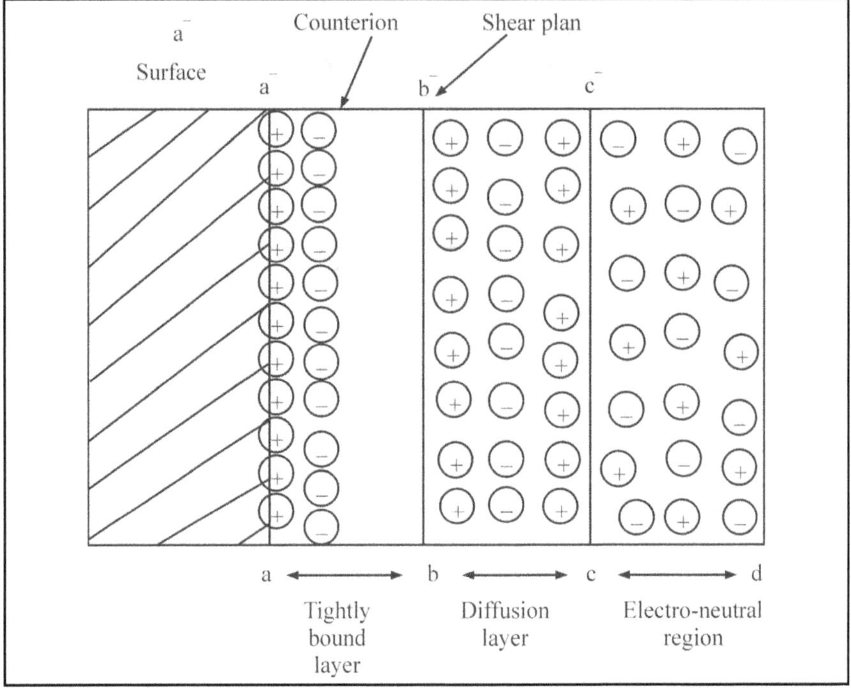

FIGURE 6.2 Electro kinetic properties.

In the above figure, the particle is positively charged and the anions present in the surrounding vehicle are attracted to the positively charged particle by electric forces that also serve to repel the approach of any cations. The ions that gave the particle its charge, cations in this example, are called potential-determining ions. Immediately adjacent to the surface of the particle is a layer of tightly bound solvent molecules, together with some ions oppositely charged to the potential-determining ions, anions in this example. These ions, oppositely charged to the potential-determining ions, are called counterions or gegenions. These two layers of ions at the interface constitute a double layer of electric charge. The intensity of the electric force decreases with distance from the surface of the particle. Thus, the distribution of ions is uniform at this region and a zone of electro neutrality is achieved.

Nernst and zeta potential: The difference in electric potential between the actual surface of the particle and the electroneutral region is referred to as Nernst potential. Thus, Nernst potential is controlled by the electrical potential at the surface of the particle due to the potential determining ions. Nernst potential has little effect in the formulation of stable suspension.

The potential difference between the ions in the tightly bound layer and the electroneutral region, referred to as zeta potential (see the figure), has significant effect in the formulation of stable suspension. Zeta potential governs the degree of repulsion between adjacent, similar charged, solid dispersed particles.

If the zeta potential is reduced below a critical value, the force of attraction between particles succeed the force of repulsion, and the particles come together. This phenomenon is referred to as flocculation and the loosely packed particles are called floccules.

6.2.5 Quality Control Tests for Suspensions

6.2.5.1 Sedimentation Volume

Sedimentation volume of a suspension is expressed by the ratio of the equilibrium volume of the sediment, V_u, to the total volume, V_o of the suspension.

$$F = \frac{V_u}{V_o}$$

The value of F normally lies between 0 - 1 for any pharmaceutical suspension. The value of F provides a qualitative knowledge about the physical stability of the suspension.

Redispersibility is the major consideration in assessing the acceptability of a suspension. The measurement of the sedimentation volume and its ease of redispersion are the most common basic evaluative procedures.

6.2.5.2 Viscosity of Phases

Stability of a suspension is solely dependent on the sedimentation rate of dispersed phase, which is dependent on the viscosity of the dispersion medium. The viscosity of the dispersion medium is measured before mixing with dispersed phase and also viscosity after mixing is determined using Brooke field viscometer. The calculated values are compared with the standard values and if any difference is found necessary corrective action are taken to get optimized viscosity.

6.2.5.3 Particle Size and Size Distribution

Size and distribution of drug particle in the dispersed phase plays a vital role in stability of final suspension. It is performed by optical microscopy, laser diffraction methods, sedimentation and Coulter counter apparatus.

6.2.5.4 pH Test

pH of the phases of suspension also contribute to stability characteristics of formulations. So pH of the different vehicles, phases of suspension, before mixing and after mixing are monitored and recorded time to time to ensure optimum pH environment being maintained.

6.2.5.5 Pourability

This test is carried out on the phases of suspension after mixing to ensure that the final preparation is pourable and will not cause any problem during filling and during handling by patient.

6.2.5.6 Zeta Potential Measurement

Value of Zeta potential reflects the future stability of suspensions so it is monitored time to time to ensure optimum zeta potential. Zeta potential is measured by either Zeta meter or using micro-electrophoresis.

6.2.6 Stability Testing

1. Appearance, colour, odour and taste
2. pH
3. Specific gravity
4. Sedimentation rate
5. Sedimentation volume
6. Zeta potential measurement
7. Compatibility with container
8. Compatibility with cap liner
9. Microscopic examination
10. Determination of crystal size
11. Determination of uniform drug distribution

6.2.7 Packaging and Storage of Suspensions

Suspension should be packed in wide mouth containers having adequate air space above the liquid. It should be stored in tight containers protected from freezing, excessive heat and light.

Label: It should be labelled as: "Shake Before Use" to ensure uniform distribution of solid particles and thereby uniform and proper dosage.

6.3 Emulsions

Emulsions are thermodynamically unstable two phase system consisting of two immiscible liquids in which one of the phase is finely subdivided and uniformly dispersed as droplets throughout the other phase.

Advantages

1. Mask the bitter taste and odour of drugs, thereby making them more palatable. *e.g.*: castor oil, cod-liver oil etc.
2. Prolong the release of the drug thereby providing sustained release action.
3. Provides protection to drugs which are susceptible to oxidation or hydrolysis.

4. Some drugs absorb faster when administered orally in the form of emulsion *e.g.* heparin

5. Patient acceptance as they are having high degree of elegance.

Disadvantages

1. Formulation needs to be shaken well before use.

2. Proper storage requires as, may affect stability.

3. Bulky and do not offer a convenient transport due to possible container breakages.

4. Liable to microbial contamination which can lead to cracking.

5. Use of a measuring device requires in order administering the accurate dose to the patient.

6.3.1 Types of Emulsions

6.3.1.1 Oil/Water and Water/Oil Emulsions

These usually have a size range of 0.1-5 μm with an average of 1-2 μm.

6.3.1.2 Multiple Emulsions

These are emulsions-of-emulsions, Water/Oil/Water, and Oil/Water/Oil systems.

6.3.1.3 Micellar Emulsions or Microemulsions

These usually have the size range of 5-50 nm. They are thermodynamically stable.

6.3.1.4 Nanoemulsions

These usually have a size range of 20-100 nm. Similar to macro-emulsions, they are only kinetically stable.

Simple emulsions are labelled as oil-in water (O/W) when they exhibit oil drops dispersed in an aqueous phase, or water-in-oil (W/O) if the opposite occurs, while multiple or double emulsions are symbolized either by W1/O/W2 or O1/W/O2. From the symbols given W1 or O1 and W2 or O2 indicate the most internal and most external phases respectively. W1 (respectively O1) and W2 (respectively O2) indicate the most internal phase and the most external one. The differentiation between these types of emulsions are shown in Table 6.9.

TABLE 6.9

Difference between O/W and W/O emulsions

S.No	Oil in water emulsion (O/W)	Water in oil emulsion (W/O)
1	Water is the dispersion medium and oil is the dispersed phase	Oil is the dispersion medium and water is the dispersed phase
2	They are non-greasy and easily removable from the skin surface	They are greasy and not water washable
3	They are used externally to provide cooling effect e.g. vanishing cream	They are used externally to prevent evaporation of moisture from the surface of skin e.g. Cold cream
4	They are preferred for formulations meant for internal use as bitter taste of oils can be masked.	They are preferred for formulations meant for external use like creams.
5	O/W emulsions give a positive conductivity test as water is the external phase which is a good conductor of electricity.	W/O emulsions do not give a positive conductivity test as oil is the external phase which is a poor conductor of electricity.

6.3.2 Tests used to Identify Emulsion Type

6.3.2.1 Dilution Test

In this test the emulsion is diluted either with oil or water. If the emulsion is o/w type and it is diluted with water, it will remain stable as water is the dispersion medium but if it is diluted with oil, the emulsion will break as oil and water are not miscible with each other.

6.3.2.2 Conductivity Test

This test is based on the basic principle that water is a good conductor of electricity. Therefore, in case of o/w emulsion, this test will be positive as water is the external phase.

6.3.2.3 Dye Solubility Test

In this test, when an emulsion is mixed with a water soluble dye such as amaranth and observed under the microscope, if the continuous phase appears red, then it means that the emulsion is o/w type as water is the external phase and the dye will dissolve in it to give colour but if the scattered globules appear red and continuous phase colourless, then it is w/o type. Similarly, if an oil soluble dye such as scarlet red C or sudan III is added to an emulsion and the continuous phase appears red, then it is w/o emulsion.

6.3.2.4 Cobalt Chloride Test

When a filter paper soaked in cobalt chloride solution is added to an emulsion and dried, it turns from blue to pink, indicating that the emulsion is o/w type and vice versa for the other type of emulsion.

6.3.2.5 Fluorescence Test

If an emulsion on exposure to ultra-violet radiations shows continuous florescence under microscope, then it is w/o type and if it shows only spotty fluorescence, then it is o/w type of emulsion.

6.3.3 Formulation of Emulsion

- *Oil Phase*: Selection of oil phase depends on the purpose of the product. Type of oil used may have effects on the viscosity of the product.

  Fixed oils of vegetable origin such as Arachis oil, sesame oil, cotton seed oil etc., are used and oils of animal origin such as cod liver oil can be used.

- *Emulsifying Agents*: These are the substances added to an emulsion to prevent the coalescence of the globules of the dispersed phase. Emulsifying agents are selected on the basis of:
  - Required shelf life stability
  - Cost
  - Type of emulsion
  - Toxicity
  - Route of administration

These agents have both a hydrophilic and a lipophilic part in their chemical structure and act in three ways:

1. *Mechanical stabilization*: Formation of a protective barrier.
2. *Thermodynamic stabilization*: Reduction of interfacial tension.
3. *Electrical stabilization*: Decreasing the potential for coalescence. by forming an electrical double layer.

Properties of Surfactants

Interfacial phenomena: Interfacial phenomena are the ones that occur at the limit between two immiscible phases, so called surface or interface. Emulsifying agents tend to be located preferentially at the interface between a polar and a nonpolar phase. The phenomenon according to which a molecule comes from the bulk of a solution to place itself at the interface (with some specific orientation) is called adsorption, and is characteristic of many amphiphilic molecules. Surfactant molecules in solution exhibits a tendency to self-associate to produce aggregation polymer called micelles, as well as other structures.

Amphiphile: An amphiphile is a chemical substance that possesses some affinity for both the polar substances and the non-polar ones and these affinities are referred to as hydrophilic and lipophilic (or hydrophobic) respectively. Most amphiphilic substances are surfactants, i.e., substances that are preferentially located at a surface or interface, where the polarity changes drastically within a few angstroms units.

Adsorption: When a surfactant molecule goes to the interface and positions itself there with some preferential orientation, it is said that the molecule is adsorbed. Adsorption is a spontaneous phenomenon which is driven by a reduction of the energy when the surfactant lyophobic group is removed from the solvent, and when one or both affinities are satisfied respectively at a surface or at an interface.

Self-Association: The second fundamental property of surfactant molecules is their capability of self-association in aqueous and non-aqueous solutions. The tendency of the surfactant molecules to associate depends upon the formation of an adsorbed monolayer, which is the first step of surfactant association. On increasing the concentration of surfactant molecules it first saturates the interface, and then accumulate in the solution. Each time a new surfactant molecule is added to the solution, the unfavorable interaction between the surfactant hydrophobic tail and the water molecules is increased. At some point the surfactant molecules start aggregating into the so-called micelles, a self-association structure in which the hydrophobic tail is removed from the aqueous environment. The concentration at which the first micelles are formed is called the Critical Micelle Concentration, which is abbreviated as CMC.

The CMC is the concentration at which the factors which favour the formation of the micelle. Micellar solutions are able to solubilize different kinds of substance, and this capacity of solubilisation is one of the most important properties of the surfactant solutions. Hydrophobic substances, i.e., oils, can be solubilized inside the micelles core, sometimes in very sizeable amounts. Some extreme cases are known in which the solubilized oil volume is actually larger than the aqueous solvent volume; for such situation to happen, the solution must contain a very large number of micelles and the micelles must be considerably swollen. These micelles are no longer spherical, but cigar shaped or hexagonally packed or even degraded into lamellar liquid crystals.

The choice of selection of emulsifying agent plays a very important role in the formulation of a stable emulsion. No single emulsifying agent possesses all the properties required for the formulation of a stable emulsion therefore sometimes blends of emulsifying agents have to be taken.

Qualities required for an ideal emulsifying agent

- It should be able to reduce the interfacial tension between the two immiscible liquids.

- It should be physically and chemically stable, inert and compatible with the other ingredients of the formulation.

- It should be completely non-irritant and nontoxic in the concentrations used.

- It should be organoleptically inert i.e., should not impart any colour, odour or taste to the preparation.

- It should be able to form a coherent film around the globules of the dispersed phase and should prevent the coalescence of the droplets of the dispersed phase.

- It should be able to produce and maintain the required viscosity of the preparation.

Classification of Emulsifying Agents

1. *Natural emulsifying agents*: A large number of emulsifiers are natural products derived from plant or animal tissue. These are hydrocolloids that form multi-molecular layers around emulsion droplets. Hydrocolloid type emulsifiers have little or no effect on interfacial tension, but exert a protective colloidal effect, reducing the potential for coalescence, by:

   - providing a protective sheath around the droplets
   - imparting a charge to the dispersed droplets (so that they repel each other)

- swelling to increase the viscosity of the system (so that droplets are less likely to merge)

Natural emulsifying agents from vegetable sources:

These consist of agents which are carbohydrates and include gums and mucilaginous substances. Since these substances are of variable chemical composition, these exhibit considerable variation in emulsifying properties. They are anionic in nature and produce o/w emulsions. They act as primary emulsifying agents and also secondary emulsifying agents (emulsion stabilizers). Since carbohydrates act as a good medium for the growth of microorganism, emulsions prepared using these emulsifying agents have to be suitably preserved in order to prevent microbial contamination. *E.g.*: tragacanth, acacia, agar, pectin and starch.

Natural emulsifying agents from animal source:

The examples include gelatin, egg yolk and wool fat (anhydrous lanolin).

2. ***Semi-synthetic polysaccharides***: Includes mainly cellulose derivatives and are used for formulating o/w type of emulsions. They are nontoxic, and are less subject to microbial growth. They primarily act by increasing the viscosity of the system. *e.g.*: Methyl cellulose, Sodium carboxymethyl cellulose etc.

3. ***Synthetic emulsifying agents***: This group contains surface active agents which act by getting adsorbed at the oil water interface in such a way that the hydrophilic polar groups are oriented towards water and lipophilic non polar groups are oriented towards oil, thus forming a stable film. This film acts as a mechanical barrier and prevents coalescence of the globules of the dispersed phase. They are classified according to the ionic charge possessed by the molecules of the surfactant *e.g.*, anionic, cationic, non-ionic and ampholytic.

  (i) ***Anionic Surfactants***: *E.g.*: Alkali soaps, amine soaps, metallic soaps, alkyl sulphates phosphates and sulphonates.

  (ii) ***Cationic surfactants***: *E.g.*: Quaternary ammonium compounds such as cetrimide, benzalkonium chloride and benzethonium chloride.

  (iii) ***Non-ionic surfactants***: *E.g.*: Glyceryl esters such as glyceryl monostearate, propylene glycol monostearate, macrogol esters such as polyoxyl stearates and polyoxyl-castor oil derivatives, sorbitan fatty acid esters such as spans and their polyoxyethylene derivatives such as tweens (polysorbates).

(iv) ***Ampholytic surfactants*:** These are the substances whose ionic charge depends on the pH of the system. Below a certain pH, these are cationic while above a defined pH, these are cationic. At intermediate pH these behave as zwitterions. *e.g.*: lecithin.

4. ***Finely divided solids*:** They accumulate at the oil/water interface and form a coherent interfacial film around the droplets of dispersed phase globules and prevent coalescence. If the solid particles are preferentially wetted by oil, a w/o emulsion is formed while if wetting is done by water then o/w emulsion is seen. *e.g.*, bentonite, aluminium magnesium stearate, attapulgite, colloidal anhydrous silica and hectorite.

5. ***Auxillary emulsifying agents*:** A variety of fatty acids (*e.g.*, stearic acid), fatty alcohols (*e.g.*, stearyl or cetyl alcohol), and fatty esters (*e.g.*, glyceryl monostearate) serve to stabilize creams through their ability to thicken the emulsion. Because these agents have only weak emulsifying properties, they are always used in combination with other emulsifiers.

Selection of Emulsifying Agents using HLB Method

A system was developed in 1949 by William C. Griffin to assist making systemic decisions about the amounts and types of surfactants needed in stable products. The system is called the HLB (hydrophile-lipophile balance) system and has an arbitrary scale of 1-18 as shown in table 6.10. HLB numbers are experimentally determined for the different emulsifiers.

TABLE 6.10

HLB system

HLB Range	USE
0-3	Antifoaming agents
4-6	W/O emulsifying agent
7-9	Wetting agents
8-18	O/W emulsifying agent
13-15	Detergents
10-18	Solubilizing agents

An emulsifier having a low HLB number indicates that the number of hydrophilic groups present in the molecule is less and it has a lipophillic character. For example, spans generally have low HLB number and they are also oil soluble. Because of their oil soluble character, spans cause the oil phase to predominate and form a w/o emulsion.

A higher HLB number indicate that the emulsifier has a large number of hydrophilic groups on the molecule and therefore is more hydrophilic in nature. Tweens have higher HLB numbers and they are also water soluble. Because of their water soluble character, tweens will cause the water phase to predominate and form an o/w emulsion.

- ***Preparation of Emulsions***: An O/W emulsion is prepared by dispersing the oily phase completely into minute globules surrounding each globule with an envelope of emulsifying agent and finally suspends the globules in the aqueous phase. Vice versa to this the W/O emulsion is prepared.

Continental and dry gum method: Emulsions are usually made by continental or dry gum method. In this method, the emulsion is prepared by mixing the emulsifying agent (usually acacia) with the oil which is then mixed with the aqueous phase. The only difference between continental and dry gum methods isthe proportion of constituents.

Wet gum method: In wet gum method, the proportion of the constituents is same as those used in the dry gum method; the only difference is the method of preparation. Here, the mucilage of the emulsifying agent (usually acacia) is formed. The oil is then added to the mucilage drop by drop with continuous trituration.

Phase inversion method: In this method, the aqueous phase is first added to the oil phase so as to form a W/O emulsion. At the point of inversion, the addition of more water results in the inversion of emulsion which gives rise to an O/W emulsion.

6.3.4 Instabilities in Emulsions

An emulsion is a thermodynamically unstable preparation due to:

Increase in surface energy caused due to the combination of interfacial tension and large surface area of the dispersed phase and difference in the densities of two phase.

Hence, care has to be taken that the chemical as well as the physical stability of the preparation remains intact throughout the shelf life. There should be no appreciable change in the mean particle size or the size distribution of the droplets of the dispersed phase and secondly droplets of the dispersed phase should remain uniformly distributed throughout the system. Signs of instability in emulsion are:

6.3.4.1 Creaming and Sedimentation

This process results from external forces usually gravitational or centrifugal forces. Under the influence of gravity suspended particles or globules tend to upward movement, known as creaming while downward movement of particles or droplets is called sedimentation. Creaming or sedimentation depends on the difference in specific gravity between the phases. Separation of an emulsion into two regions, one phase which is richer in dispersed phase than the other, but remains in the form of globules, which may be redistributed throughout the dispersion medium by shaking. Increasing the viscosity of the medium decreases the tendency to cream. Creaming is a reversible phenomenon which can be corrected by mild shaking. The factors affecting creaming are best described by stokes law

$$V = 2r^2 (d_1 - d_2) \frac{g}{9n}$$

where V = rate of creaming

     r = radius of globules

     d_1 = density of dispersed phase

     d_2 = density of dispersion medium

     g = gravitational constant

     n = viscosity of the dispersion medium

The following approaches can be used for decreasing creaming:

- *Globule size*: According to stokes law, rate of creaming is directly proportional to the size of globules. Bigger is the size of the globules, more will be the creaming. Therefore, in order to minimize creaming, globule size should be reduced by homogenization.

- *Viscosity*: Rate of creaming is inversely proportional to the viscosity of the continuous phase i.e. more the viscosity of the continuous phase less will the problem of creaming. Therefore, to avoid creaming in emulsions, the viscosity of the continuous phase should be increased by adding suitable viscosity enhancers like gum acacia, tragacanth etc.

- **Density**: Less difference in density of two phases means more stability of emulsion.

- **Temperature**: Lower temperature is more suitable for the better stability of emulsion

6.3.4.2 Flocculation

Flocculation is a reversible aggregation of droplets of the internal phase in the form of three dimensional clusters within the emulsion. Particle droplet comes together but does not fuse and individual droplets retain their identities but each cluster behaves physically as a single discrete unit.

6.3.4.3 Cracking (Coalescence)

It is a process by which emulsified particles fuse together to form large particle. Complete fusion of the droplets occurs and total surface free energy decreases as surface area increases. Cracking of emulsion can be due to addition of an incompatible emulsifying agent, chemical or microbial decomposition of emulsifying agent, addition of electrolytes, exposure to increased or reduced temperature or change in pH.

6.3.4.4 Phase Inversion

In phase inversion o/w type emulsion changes into w/o type and vice versa. It is a physical instability. It may be brought about by the addition of an electrolyte or by changing the phase volume ratio or by temperature changes. The temperature at which the inversion occurs depends on the emulsifier concentration and is called phase inversion temperature. An o/w emulsion is stabilized by a non-ionic polyoxyethylene derived surfactant. Phase inversion can be minimized by using the proper emulsifying agent in adequate concentration, keeping the concentration of dispersed phase between 30 to 60 % and by storing the emulsion in a cool place.

6.3.4.5 Ostwald Ripening (Disproportionation)

This results from the finite solubility of the liquid phases. Ostwald ripening causes the diffusion of monomers from smaller to larger droplets due to greater solubility of the single monomer molecules in the larger monomer droplets. With time, the smaller droplets disappear and their molecules diffuse to the bulk and become deposited on the larger droplets. This can lead to the destabilization of emulsions (creaming and sedimentation).

The result of such a process is smaller particles get smaller, while the larger ones get even larger i.e. Growth of large particles at expense of small ones. The rate of Ostwald ripening is determined by concentration gradient around the particles, the latter is in turn dependent on the particles size

6.3.5 Packaging, Labelling and Storage of Emulsions

Depending on the use, emulsions should be packed in suitable containers. Emulsions meant for oral use are usually packed in well filled bottles having an air tight closure. Light sensitive products are packed in amber coloured bottles. For viscous emulsions, wide mouth bottles should be used.

Comply with general requirements for labeling, in addition the label should indicate following information: quantity of emulsifying agent, preservative, "Shake well before use", and "Keep in cool place" External use products should clearly mention on their label that they are meant for external use only

Preservation from micro organisms: It is necessary to preserve the emulsions from microorganisms as these can proliferate easily in emulsified systems with high water content, particularly if carbohydrates, proteins or steroidal materials are also present.

Contamination due to microorganisms can result in problems such as colour and odour change, gas production, hydrolysis, pH change and eventually breaking of emulsion. Therefore, is necessary that emulsified systems be adequately preserved. An ideal preservative should be non-irritant, non-sensitizing and nontoxic in the concentration used. It should be physically as well as chemically compatible with other ingredients of the emulsions and with the proposed container of the product. It should not impart any taste, colour or odour to the product. It should be stable and effective over a wide range of pH and temperature. It should have a wide spectrum of activity against a range of bacteria, yeasts and moulds. The selective preservative should have high water solubility and a low oil/water partition coefficient. It should have bactericidal rather than bacteriostatic activity.

Examples of antimicrobial preservatives used to preserve emulsified systems include parahydroxybenzoate esters such as methyl, propyl and butyl parabens, organic acids such as ascorbic acid and benzoic acid, organic mercurials such as phenylmercuric acetate and phenylmercuric nitrate, quarternary ammonium compounds such as cetrimide, cresol derivatives such as chlorocresol and miscellaneous agents such as sodium benzoate, chloroform and phenoxyethanol.

Preservation from oxidation: Oxidative changes such as rancidity and spoilage due to atmospheric oxygen and effects of enzymes produced by micro-organisms is seen in many emulsions containing vegetables, mineral oils and animal fats. Antioxidants can be used to prevent the changes occurring due to atmospheric oxygen.

Antioxidants are agents having a high affinity for oxygen and compete for it with labile substances in the formulation. The ideal antioxidant should be nontoxic, nonirritant, effective at low concentration under the expected conditions of storage and use, soluble in the medium and stable. Antioxidants for use in oral preparation should also be odourless and tasteless.

Some of the commonly used anti-oxidants for emulsified systems include alkyl gallate such as ethyl, propyl or dodecyl gallate, butylated hydroxyanisole (BH), butylated hydroxytoluene (BHT)

6.3.6 Quality Control Tests for Emulsions

The following are the quality control tests done for emulsions:

6.3.6.1 Particle Size and Particle Size Distribution

It is performed by optical microscopy, sedimentation and Coulter counter apparatus.

6.3.6.2 Determination of Viscosity

Determination of viscosity is done to assess the changes that might take place during aging. The viscometers which should be used include cone and plate viscometers. For viscous emulsions, the use of penetrometer is used.

6.3.6.3 Phase Separation Determination

Phase separation may be observed visually or by measuring the volume of the separated phases.

6.3.6.4 Electrophoretic Properties Determination

Zeta potential is an important parameter used for assessing emulsion stability, since electric charges on the particles affect the rate of flocculation

6.3.7 Stability Testing

Stability of emulsions is an important parameter for the formulator. Stability testing of emulsions involves determining stability at long term storage conditions, accelerated storage conditions, freezing and thawing conditions. Stress conditions are applied in order to speed up the stability testing. The stress conditions used for speeding up instability of emulsions include: Centrifugal force, agitational force, aging and temperature. The following physical parameters are evaluated to assess the effect of any of the above stress conditions:

- Phase separation
- Viscosity
- Electrophoretic properties
- Particle size and particle number

Typical test programme for assessment of stability:

1. Emulsion should be stable with no visible sign of separation for at least

   - 60-90 days at 45-50 °C
   - 5-6 months at 37 °C
   - 12-18 month at room temperature

2. There should be no visible sign of separation after one-month storage at 4 °C and 2-3 °C freeze thaw cycles between –20 °C and 25 °C

3. Emulsion should survive at least 6-8 heating/cooling cycle between refrigeration temperature and 45 °C of not less than 48 hours.

4. A stable emulsion should show no deterioration by centrifuge at 2000-3000 rpm at room temperature.

5. Emulsion should not be adversely affected by agitation for 24-48 hours on a reciprocating shaker.

6.3.8 Dry Emulsions

Dry emulsions present a potential oral drug delivery system for lipophilic and low soluble drug substances and for drug substances needing protection against light. These are of prime importance due to its stability and sustained release effect.

For the preparation of dry emulsions, we require drug, solid carrier, aqueous phase and lipophilic solvent. The solid carriers used to prepare dry emulsions are gelatin, lactose, maltodextrin, mannitol, povidone, sucrose and colloidal silica. Dry emulsions can be prepared by spray drying, lyophilization and rotary evaporation.

6.3.9 Microemulsions

Microemulsions are thermodynamically stable clear, optically transparent isotropic mixtures of biphasic oil, water and surfactant. They contain globules having a diameter ranging from 0.1 to 100 micrometers.

Advantages

- Spontaneous formation
- Ease of manufacturing and scale-up
- Thermodynamic stability
- Improved drug solubilisation
- Enhancement of bioavailability
- More rapid and efficient absorption
- Transparency
- Stability.

Disadvantages

- Requires large quantity of surfactant
- The possibility of disruption of the crystalline structure of stratum corneum, which leads to skin irritation
- Prone to phase separation.

Applications: Microemulsions have been promisingly used as drug delivery system for its advantages including their thermodynamic stability, optical clarity, improving the efficacy of a drug and ease of penetration. Microemulsions are potential drug carrier systems for oral, topical, and parenteral administration. Microemulsions are simple and convenient novel vehicles for delivery of medicaments which can enhance drug absorption with reduced systemic side effects.

- ***Drug Targeting***: By altering pharmacokinetics and bio-distribution of drugs and restricting their action to the targeted tissue increased drug efficacy with concomitant reduction of their toxic effects can be achieved by microemulsion deliveries. Microemulsion formulation for tumour targeting of lipophilic antitumor antibiotic aclainomycin A.

- ***Cellular Targeting***: Nucleic acids delivered to cells are promising therapeutics. A recent research included insertion of nucleic acid into a reverse micelle (Microemulsion) for cell delivery

- ***Tumour Targeting***: Microemulsions used as vehicles for the delivery of chemotherapeutic or diagnostic agents to neoplastic cells while avoiding normal cells.

- ***Ocular and Pulmonary Delivery***: O/W microemulsions have been investigated for ocular administration, to dissolve poorly soluble drugs, to increase absorption and to attain prolonged release profile.

6.3.10 Multiple Emulsions

Multiple emulsions are also called as "emulsion of emulsion". These are complex systems in which the O/W or W/O emulsions are dispersed in another liquid medium. There are mainly two types of multiple emulsions O/W/O and W/O/W emulsions. O/W/O emulsion consists of very small droplets of oil dispersed in the water globules of a W/O emulsion and a W/O/W emulsion consists of droplets of water dispersed in the oil phase of an O/W.

Preparation of Multiple Emulsion

- ***Phase Inversion Technique or Single Step Technique***: The method involves the addition of an aqueous phase containing the hydrophilic emulsifier (Tween 80/Sodium Docedyl Sulphate) to an oil phase consisted of liquid paraffin and containing liophillic emulsifier (Span 80).

- ***Two-Step Emulsification***: This method involves re-emulsification of primary W/O or O/W emulsion using a suitable emulsifying agents. The first step involves the preparation of primary emulsions which is then re-emulsified with an excess of aqueous phase or oil phase in the presence of second emulsifier. An aqueous solution of emulsifier is then introduced successively to the oil phase in the vessel at a rate of 5 Ml/min, while the pin mixer rotates steadily at 88 rpm at room temperature. When volume fraction of the aqueous solution of hydrophilic emulsifier exceeds 0.7, the continuous oil phase is substituted by the aqueous phase containing a number of the vesicular globules among the simple oil droplets, leading to phase inversion and formation of W/O/W multiple emulsion.

- ***Membrane Emulsification Technique:*** This method uses low shear forces to produce emulsions. A W/O emulsion is extruded into an external aqueous phase with a constant pressure through a Porous Glass Membrane, which should have controlled and homogenous pores. The droplets formed at the membrane surface are detached by the continuous external aqueous phase flowing across the membrane surface. To support the emulsification and prevent coalescence of droplets, a surface active compound must be added to the continuous phase It can be successfully applied to make multiple emulsions as drug delivery systems

Advantages

- Mask the bitter taste and odour of drugs, thus making them more palatable. *e.g.*: Castor oil, Chloroquine Phosphate etc.
- Biocompatible.
- Prolong the release of the drug.
- Protection to drugs which are susceptible to oxidation or hydrolysis.
- Enhancing oral bioavailability or oral absorption.

Disadvantages

- Thermodynamically instable.
- Short shelf life.
- Complex structure.

Pharmaceutical Applications: Multiple emulsions have significant applications in food, agricultural, pharmaceutical, and cosmetic industries in which they can facilitate the sustained release and transport of active material. These are also applied in:

- Taste masking
- Vaccine adjuvant
- Enzyme immobilization
- Drug over dosage treatment/detoxification

- Controlled and Sustained Drug Delivery
- Drug targeting to tumour cells.

Multiple emulsions have been formulated as cosmetics, such as skin moisturizer. Prolonged release can also be obtained by means of multiple emulsions.

Some Industrial Formulations

1. Abacavir Sulfate Oral Solution

Formulation

Material name	Quantity/L (g)
Abacavir, use abacavir hemisulfate	23.40
Sorbitol 70%	344.40
Sodium saccharin	0.30
Strawberry flavour	2.00
Banana flavour	2.00
Sodium citrate dehydrate for pH adjustment	10.00
Citric acid anhydrous for pH adjustment	7.00
Methyl paraben	1.50
Propyl paraben	0.18
Propylene glycol	50.00
Hydrochloric acid dilute for pH adjustment to 4.0	q.s.
Sodium hydroxide for pH adjustment	q.s.

Manufacturing Directions

1. The pH range for this solution is from 3.8 to 4.5.
2. Charge 40% of the propylene glycol to an appropriately sized stainless steel container and add methyl paraben and propylparaben with mixing, and mix until dissolved.
3. Charge purified water into a stainless steel manufacturing tank equipped with a suitable mixer to approximately 40% of final batch volume.
4. Add sorbitol solution to the manufacturing tank.
5. While mixing, add item 1 and mix until dissolved.
6. While continuing to mix the paraben/glycol solution, the remaining propyleneglycol, artificial strawberry flavour, artificial banana

flavour, saccharin sodium, citric acid anhydrous, and sodium citrate dihydrate are added and mixed until dissolved.

7. Turn off the mixer and bring the solution to a volume of 500 L, and mix until a homogeneous solution is achieved.

8. Measure and adjust pH to 3.8 to 4.5 with sodium hydroxide or hydrochloric acid.

9. Filter the solution through a clarifying filter into an appropriately sized receiving vessel.

2. Acetaminophen Oral Suspension

Material name	Quantity/L (g)
Acetaminophen micronized, 2.0% excess	51.00
Sucrose	500.00
Methyl paraben	1.00
Propyl paraben	0.30
Sodium citrate	0.06
Glycerin (Glycerol)	7.00
Sorbitol (70%)	80.00
Xanthan gum (Keltrol F)	400.00
Dye	2.00
Flavour	0.10
Strawberry flavour	0.70
Water purified	q.s. to 1 L

Manufacturing Directions

1. Acetaminophen dispersion should be uniformly mixed or levigated. If acetaminophen dispersion is either added to hot syrup base or homogenized for a long time, flocculation may appear. While handling the syrup, mucilage, or drug dispersion, the handling loss should not be more than 1%. If the loss exceeds 1%, it may give poor suspension.

2. Add 180 g of item13 to the mixer and heat to 90 °C.

3. Dissolve items 3 and item 4 while mixing. Add and dissolve item 2 while mixing. Cool down to about 50^0 to 55 °C.

4. Add and dissolve item 5 while mixing. Filter the syrup through T 1500 filters washed withitem13. Collect the syrup in clean stainless steel tank.

5. Disperse item 9 in item 6 in a separate stainless steel container. Add 40 g of hot item 13 (90 °C) at once while mixing. Mix for 20 minutes to make a homogeneous smooth mucilage.

6. Mix item 7 in 10 g of item 13 (25 °C) in a separate stainless steel container. Add item 1while mixing with stirrer. Mix for 25 minutes to make uniform suspension.

7. Add sugar syrup and mucilage to the mixer. Rinse the container of mucilage with 15 g of item 13 and add the rinsing to the mixer. Cool to 25 °C while mixing.

8. Add item 1 dispersion to the mixer. Rinse the container of dispersion with 15 g of item 13and add rinsing to the mixer. Check the suspension for uniformity of dispersion.

9. Mix for additional 5 minutes at 18 rpm, vacuum0.5 bar if required.

10. Add item 8 to the mixer and mix for 10 minutes. Dissolve item 10 in 7 g of item 13 and add to the mixer.

11. Disperse item 11 in 7 g of item 13 and add to the mixer. Add item 12 to the mixer.

12. Add cold item 13 (25 °C) to make up the volume up to 1.0 L.

13. Homogenize for 5 minutes at low speed under vacuum 0.5 bar, 18 rpm, temperature 25 °C.

14. Check the dispersion for uniformity.

15. Check the pH. Limit 5.7 ± 0.5 at 25.C. If required adjust the pH with 20% solution of citric Acid or Sodium Citrate.

16. Transfer the suspension through 630-micronsieve after mixing for 5 minutes at 18-20 rpm, temperature NMT 25 °C, to the stainless steel storage tank.

3. Acetaminophen Syrup for Children

Material name	Quantity/L (g)
Acetaminophen, crystalline	25.00
Kollidon 25 or Kollidon 30	300.00
Glycerol	600.00
Sodium cyclamate	40.00
Orange flavour	<01.0
Raspberry flavour	2.00
Water	575.00

Manufacturing Directions

1. Dissolve Kollidon in water, add acetaminophen and sodium cyclamate, heat to 50 °C, and stir to obtain a clear solution.

2. Dissolve the flavours and mix with glycerol. The obtained syrup is a viscous, clear, sweet, and only slightly bitter liquid.

4. Acyclovir Oral Suspension

Material Name	Quantity/L (g)
Acyclovir	43.00
Methyl paraben	1.00
Propyl paraben	0.20
Microcrystalline cellulose (Avicel RC – 591)	15.00
Glycerine (glycerol)	150.00
Sorbitol (70% solution)	450.00
Orange/banana dry flavour	4.00
Water, purified	q.s. to 1 L

Manufacturing Directions

1. Disperse item 1 in item 6. Keep stirring by stirrer for 1 hour.

2. Heat 333.33 g of item 8 in mixer to 90 °C to 95 °C. Dissolve items 2 and 3 while mixing. Cool to30 °C.

3. Disperse items 4 and 5 in a stainless steel container and keep stirring for 1 hour.

4. Add step 3 into step 2 at 30 °C. Mix and homogenize for 5 minutes at high speed under vacuum 0.5 bar.

5. Add step 1 in to step 2 and mix for 5 minutes.

6. Disperse item 7 in 13.33 g of item 8. Add into step 2.

7. Make up the volume with item

8. Finally, homogenize for 5 minutes at high speed under vacuum 0.5 bar.

Recent advancements in Liquid Dosage Form

Suspension

- *Micro/ Nano Suspension*: Micro/Nano suspension consists of the pure poorly water-soluble drug without any matrix material suspended in dispersion. Micro/Nano suspension increases dissolution rate and absorption of drug due to smaller particle size and larger surface area. Micro/Nano suspensions are used in oral, parenteral, ocular delivery of the drugs for sustained release.

- ***Taste Masked Suspension*****:** Used to mask bitter taste of drugs.

- ***Sustained release Suspension*****:** API in suspended form control the rate of release as well as maintaining desire drug level in the blood for long duration.

- ***Dry Suspension*****:** Dry suspension is dry mixtures that require addition of water at the time of dispensing.

Emulsion

- ***Multiple Emulsion*****:** Multiple emulsion are used for prolonged action, Target delivery, taste masking, improved stability, enzyme entrapment, protection against external environment.

- ***Micro/Nano Emulsion*****:** It offers advantages as fast onset of action, better bioavailability, and stability than conventional emulsion. Nanoemulsion formulations have distinct advantages over macro emulsion systems when delivered parenterally because of the small particle size.

- ***Liposome Emulsion*****:** Liposomal Emulsion are used for drug targeting safely to its target site in the precise time period to have a controlled release and attain the maximum therapeutic effect

- ***Dry Emulsion*****:** Dry emulsions are lipid based powder formulations from which an emulsion can be reconstituted. The dry emulsion formulation improves the bioavailability of drug substances and reduces their side effects. These are physically and microbiologically stable formulations and represent a potential oral drug delivery system for lipophilic and low soluble drug substances.

- ***Non Aqueous Emulsion*****:** Non-aqueous systems are well known as solvents for drugs, suspension vehicles, and oleo gels.

- ***Gellified emulsion* (*Emulsion in gel*):** Have emerged as one of the most interesting topical drug delivery system as it has dual release control system i.e., emulsion and gel.

- ***Self-Emulsifying Drug Delivery Systems*** **(SEDDS):** It is a drug delivery system that uses a microemulsion achieved by chemical rather than mechanical mean. These multi component delivery systems have the ability to self-emulsify when introduced to an aqueous medium under gentle agitation.

7 Semisolid Dosage Forms

7.1 Introduction

Semisolids constitute an important section of pharmaceutical dosage forms. They serve as carriers for drugs that are topically delivered by route of the skin, rectal tissue, nasal mucosal, vaginal, buccal tissue, urethral membrane, and external ear lining. Semi-solid dosage forms are normally presented in the form of creams, gels, ointments, or pastes. They contain one or more active ingredients dissolved or uniformly dispersed in a suitable base and any suitable excipients such as emulsifiers, viscosity-increasing agents, antimicrobial agents, antioxidants, or stabilizing agents.

7.1.1 Topical Drug Delivery

Topical preparations are applied to the skin or mucus membrane for medicinal or non medicinal effect. In some cases, the base may be used alone for its therapeutic properties, such as emollient, soothing or protective action.

Advantages of topical drug delivery systems

- Avoidance of first pass metabolism.
- Convenient and easy to apply.
- Avoidance of the risks and inconveniences of intravenous therapy and of the varied conditions of absorption, like pH changes, presence of enzymes, gastric emptying time etc.
- Prompt termination of the medications, when needed.
- Provides a large surface area.
- Ability to deliver drug more selectively to a specific site.
- Improve patient compliance.
- Self-medication.

Disadvantages of Topical Drug Delivery Systems

- Skin irritation of contact dermatitis may occur due to the drug and/or excipients.
- Poor permeability of some drugs through the skin.
- Possibility of allergenic reactions.
- Can be used only for drugs which require very small plasma concentration for action.
- Enzyme in epidermis may denature the drugs.
- Drugs of larger particle size are not easily absorbed through the skin.

7.1.2 Transdermal Delivery Systems

These are self-contained, discrete dosage forms designed to deliver the drug(s) through the skin to the systemic circulation.

7.1.3 Percutaneous Absorption

The absorption of drug substance from outside the skin to position beneath the skin including entrance in to the blood stream.

7.2 Anatomy and Physiology of the Skin

Most of topical preparations are meant to be applied to the skin. So basic knowledge of skin and its physiology, function and biochemistry are very important for designing transdermal formulations. Skin is the largest multilayered organ that in average weighs about 8 pounds. The skin is composed of several layers including stratum corneum, viable epidermis and dermis, and it contains appendages that include sweat glands, sebaceous glands, and hair follicles as shown in Figure 7.1. The stratum corneum is the outermost desquamating 'horny' layer of skin, comprising about 15-20 rows of flat, partially desiccated, dead, keratinized epidermal cells.

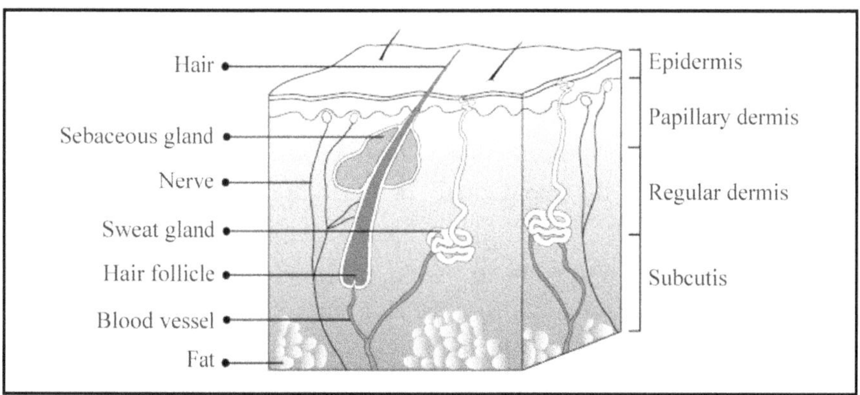

FIGURE 7.1 Anatomy and physiology of skin.

- ***Epidermis***: It is the outermost layer of the skin, which is approximately 150 micrometers thick. The outermost epidermis is made up of stratified squamous epithelium with an underlying basement membrane. It contains no blood vessels, and is nourished by diffusion from the dermis. Cells are formed through mitosis at the innermost layers. They move up the strata changing shape and composition as they differentiate and become filled with keratin. They eventually reach the corneum and become sloughed off. This process is called keratinization and takes place within about 30 days. This layer of skin is responsible for keeping water in the body and keeping other harmful chemicals and pathogens out. Blood capillaries are found beneath the epidermis

- ***Dermis***: The dermis lies below the epidermis and contains a number of structures including blood vessels, nerves, hair follicles, smooth muscle, glands and lymphatic tissue. The dermis can be split into the papillary and reticular layers. The papillary layer is outermost and extends into the dermis to supply it with vessels. It is composed of loosely arranged fibers.

- ***Hypodermis***: The hypodermis is not a part of the skin, and lies below the dermis. It is made up of loose connective tissue and elastin.

Sebaceous glands

These glands are derived from epidermal cells and are associated with hair follicles of the scalp, face, chest and back. They are small in children, enlarging and becoming active at puberty. Sebum play a role in:

- maintaining the epidermal permeability barrier, structure and differentiation
- skin-specific hormonal signalling
- transporting antioxidants to the skin surface
- Protection from UV radiation.

Sweat glands

There are about 2.5 million on the skin surface and they are present over the majority of the body. They are located within the dermis and are composed of coiled tubes, which secrete a watery substance. They are classifed into two different types: eccrine and apocrine. Eccrine glands are found all over the skin especially on the palms, soles, axillae and forehead. Apocrine glands are larger, the ducts of which empty out into the hair follicles. They are present in the axillae, anogenital region and areolae

7.3   Route of Absorption

Semisolid dosage forms for dermatological drug therapy are intended to produce desired therapeutic action at specific sites in the epidermal tissue. A drug's ability to penetrate the skin's epidermis, dermis, and subcutaneous fat layers depends on the physicochemical properties of the drug, the carrier base and skin condition. Both topical and transdermal drug products are intended for external use. However, topical dermatologic products are intended for localized action on one or more layers of the skin. When a drug system is applied topically, the drug diffuses out of its vehicle on to the surface tissue of the skin.

There are three potential portals of entry as shown in Figure 7.2.

1. Through the unbroken stratum corneum
2. Through the sweat ducts
3. Through the follicular region

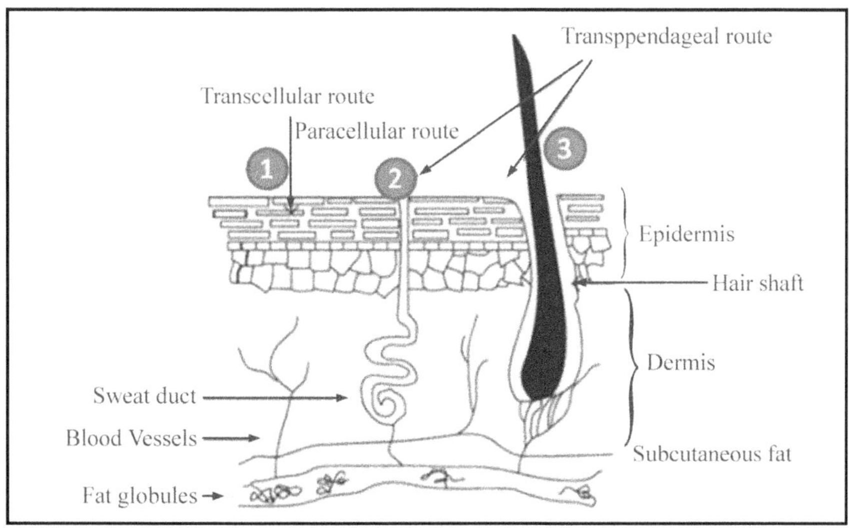

FIGURE 7.2 Routes of penetration.

7.4   Factors Affecting Skin Penetration

The factors that influence skin penetration are essentially the same as those for gastro intestinal absorption, with the rate of diffusion depending primarily on the physicochemical property of the drug and secondarily on the vehicle, pH, and concentration. Generally, drug absorption into the skin occurs by passive diffusion. The rate of drug transport across the stratum corneum follows Fick's Law of Diffusion,

$$\frac{dA}{dt} = \frac{D.A.K.\Delta C}{h}$$

.....(7.1)

where,

$\dfrac{dA}{dt}$ - steady-state flux across stratum corneum

D - the diffusion coefficient or diffusivity of drug molecules

ΔC - drug concentration gradient across the stratum corneum

K - partition coefficient of the drug between skin and formulation medium,

h - thickness of the stratum corneum

The principle physicochemical factor in skin penetration is the hydration state of stratum corneum, which affects the rate of passage of all substances that penetrate the skin. The temperature of skin and the concentration of the drug play significant roles. The solubility of a drug determines the concentration presented to the absorption site, and the water or lipid partition coefficient influences the rate of transportation. An inverse relationship appears to exist between the absorption rate and the molecular weight. Small molecules penetrate more rapidly than large molecules, but within a narrow range of molecular size, there is little correlation between the size and the penetration rate.

7.5   Functions of Skin

1. *Protection*: Skin forms an anatomical barrier against physical chemical and microbial attack.
2. *Sensation*: It contains a variety of nerve endings that react to heat, cold, touch, pressure, vibration, and tissue injury.
3. *Heat regulation*: The skin contains sebaceous glands and smooth erector pili muscles.
4. *Storage*: It acts as a storage centre for lipids and water, as well as a means of synthesis of vitamin D by action of UV rays from sun on certain parts of the skin.
5. *Temperature regulation*: by sweating.

7.6   Classification of Semisolid Dosage Forms

The topical dosage forms are classified on the basis of state is shown in Table 7.1.

TABLE 7.1

Class of topical dosage forms based on state

Types of topical preparation	Examples
Solid	• Powders, Plasters
Liquid	• Solutions, Suspensions, Emulsions
Semi solid	• Lotions, Liniments, Ointments, Creams, Pastes, Gels, Jellies, Suppositories
Gaseous	• Aerosols, Sprays

- **Ointments (Semisolid Solution):** They are soft hydrocarbon based semisolid preparation intended for external application to the skin or mucous. These are composed of fluid hydrocarbon meshed in a matrix of higher melting solid hydrocarbon petrolatum. Since they are greasy in nature they form stains.

- **Creams (Semisolid Emulsion):** Creams are semisolid dosage forms that contain one or more drug substances dissolved or dispersed in a suitable base that are water washable and more cosmetically and aesthetically acceptable. They are viscous semisolid emulsion system with opaque appearance as contrasted with translucent ointments. Consistency and rheological characters depend on whether the cream is w/o or o/w.

- **Pastes (Semisolid Suspension):** Pastes are semisolid dosage forms that contain a high percentage of finely dispersed solids with a stiff consistency and are intended for topical application. Pastes are less penetrating, less greasy and less macerating than ointments. Pastes make particularly good protective barrier.

- **Gels (Jellies):** Gels are semisolid system in which a liquid phase is constrained within a 3-D polymeric matrix consisting of natural or synthetic gum having a high degree of physical or chemical cross-linking. When the gel mass consists of a network of small discrete particles, the gel is classified as a two-phase system. In a two-phase system, if the particle size of the dispersed phase is relatively large, the gel mass is sometimes referred to as magma gels which are richer in liquid than magma. Both gels and magmas may be thixotropic, forming semisolids after standing and becoming liquid when agitated.

- **Lotions:** Lotions usually are fluids, a little viscid emulsion dosage forms for external application on the skin.

- **Poultices:** It is soft, viscous, pasty preparation for external use. They are applied to skin while they are hot. Poultice must retain heat for a considerable time because they are intended to supply warmth to inflamed parts of body.

- **Plasters:** Plasters are solid or semisolid mass adhere to the skin when spread upon cotton or felt line or muslin as a backing material and they are mainly used for protection and mechanical support.

- **Rigid Foams:** Foams are emulsified systems packaged in pressurized containers or special dispensing devices in which air or some other gas is emulsified in liquid phase.

- **Topical Aerosol:** Topical aerosols are products that are packaged under pressure. The active ingredients are released in the form of fine liquid droplets or fine powder particles upon activation of an appropriate valve system.

- **Topical Solution:** Topical solutions are liquid preparations that are usually aqueous but often contain other solvents such as alcohol and polyols that contain one or more dissolved chemical substances intended for topical application to the skin or oral mucosal surface.

- **Topical Suspension:** Topical suspensions are liquid preparations that contain solid particles dispersed in a liquid vehicle intended for application to the skin.

7.7   Formulation of Semisolid Dosage Forms

7.7.1 Ingredients used in Preparation of Semisolids

Ingredients used for formulating of semisolids include drug, bases, antimicrobial preservatives, chelating agents, humectants, fragrances.

7.7.1.1 Ointment Bases

A large number of drugs for external use are presented as semi-solid formulations *e.g.*: ointments, suppositories, creams and pastes. While ointments are considered as semi-solids, suppositories are regarded as molded solid dosage forms. Ointment and suppository bases do not only act as the carriers of the medicaments, but they also control the extent of absorption of medicaments incorporated in them.

An ointment base should be compatible with skin, stable, smooth and pliable, non-irritating, non-sensitizing, inert, capable of absorbing water or other liquid preparations, and of releasing the incorporated medicament, readily. A base for ophthalmic ointments must be non-irritating to the eye, should permit the diffusion of the drug through the secretions bathing the eye, and should retain the activity of the medicament for a reasonable period often under proper storage conditions. It should also be sterilizable conveniently.

The criteria of selection of ointment base depends on:

(i)   Desired release rate of the drug substance from the ointment base.

(ii) Rate and extent of topical or percutaneous drug absorption.

(iii) Desirability of occlusion of moisture from skin.

(iv) Stability of the drug in the ointment base.

 (v) Effect of drug on the consistency of base.

(vi) Easy removal of base on washing.

(vii) Characteristics of the surface to which it is applied.

Ointment bases may be classified in several ways but the following classification is based on compositions generally used which are as follow:

(A) Oleaginous bases

(B) Absorption bases

(C) Emulsifying bases

(D) Water removable bases

(E) Water soluble bases

A. **Oleaginous bases:** Oleaginous bases are also termed as hydrocarbon bases. These bases generally consist of a combination of more than one oleaginous material such as water-insoluble hydrophobic oils, fats and hydrocarbons derived from petroleum. Combinations of these materials can produce a wide range of melting points and viscosities. They can remain on the skin for relatively long periods without drying, and because of their immiscibility with water are difficult to wash off. White Ointment, USP is a typical combination of hydrocarbons.

- **Petrolatum:** Petrolatum is a tasteless, odorless, yellowish, greasy solid with a melting point between 38 °C and 60 °C. White petrolatum is decolorized petrolatum. It is used more frequently than yellow petrolatum. Petrolatum is very stable, very compatible with most substances, and emollient to the skin. The consistency can easily be varied by the incorporation of mineral oil or white wax. Petrolatum-type ointment bases are more stable than vegetable- or animal-type bases. However, all of these bases are greasy. The degree to which they release the incorporated medication is questionable. They are able to absorb only very small amounts of water, unless treated with cholesterol.

- **Mineral oil (Liquid petrolatum):** These are liquid hydrocarbon derived from petroleum.

- **White Ointment:** It is a typical combination of petrolatum with 5% beeswax.

B.   **Absorption bases:** They are called as emulsion bases because they initially contain no water but are capable of taking it up to yield W/O and O/W emulsions. Absorption bases are W/O type emulsions and have capacity to absorb considerable quantities of water or aqueous solution without marked changes in consistency. Absorption bases are mostly mixtures of animal sterols with petrolatum. Combinations of cholesterol and/or other suitable lanolin fractions with white petrolatum are available

- **Anhydrous bases:** These type of bases are able to absorb water to form W/O emulsion while retaining its semisolid consistency. *e.g.*: *Anhydrous lanolin.*

- **Hydrophilic petrolatum:** Aquaphore is refined variation which can absorb 3 times as weight of water. The formula is given *in* Table 7.2.

TABLE 7.2

Composition of hydrophilic petrolatum

Sr. No.	Composition	% w/v
1	Cholesterol	3
2	Stearyl alcohol	3
3	White wax	8
4	White petrolatum	86

Advantages: Highly compatible, stable, good emollients.

Disadvantages: Difficult to remove from skin and clothing.

C.   **Emulsifying bases**: According to the type of emulsion, these bases are W/O. All W/O emulsions are not water-washable as the oil is in the external phase

- **Hydrous lanolin (hydrous wool fat):** Obtained as a fat like substance from wool of sheep containing 20-30% of water.

- **Cold cream:** contain combination of borax, beeswax and mineral oil.

Advantages: These are washable and non-greasy if oil-in-water (o/w) type.

Disadvantages: These bases are subjected to water loss if o/w, greasy and not washable if water-in-oil (w/o), unless, a preservative is added, the emulsion bases are subject to mold growth.

D. Water removable bases: These are O/W type of emulsion which are commonly referred as vanishing creams.

- **Vanishing creams:** They are oil in water type creams which when rubbed onto the skin disappear with little or no trace of their former presence.

These bases are easily washable from the skin due to their hydrophilic nature and may be diluted with water or aqueous solution.

e.g.: Hydrophilic ointment (Table 7.3)

TABLE 7.3

Composition of hydrophilic ointment

Sr. No.	Composition	% w/v
1	SLS	1
2	Stearyl alcohol	25
3	White petrolatum	25
4	Propylene glycol	12
5	Purified water	37

E. Water soluble bases: These are also known as greaseless bases which are completely water washable. They are water soluble, nonvolatile, and do not deteriorate or support mold growth. They do not hydrolyse. They have low irritancy. A variety of water washable ointment bases with consistencies ranging from semi-solid to solid can be obtained by blending different polyethylene glycols. Polyethylene glycol ointment USP is a blend of carbowaxes 4000 and 400. At room temperature, carbowaxes 200 to 400 are clear liquids whereas carbowaxes greater than 1000 are white, waxy solids.

7.7.1.2 Emulsifying Agents

Ideal properties of emulsifier:

- Must reduce surface tension for proper emulsification.
- Ability to increase the viscosity at low concentration.
- Effective at low concentration.

The different types of emulsifiers are given in Table 7.4

TABLE 7.4

Types of emulsifiers

Anionic	Cationic	Nonionic
Alkyl sulphates	Quaternary ammonium compounds	Polyoxyethylene alkyl-aryl ethers
Soaps	Alkoxy alkylamines	Polyoxyethylene fatty acid ester
Dodecyl benzene sulfonate		Polyoxyethylene sorbitan esters
Lactylates		Sorbitan fatty acid esters
Sulfosuccinates		Glyceryl fatty acid esters
Monoglyceride sulfonates		Sucrose fatty acid esters
Phosphate ester		Polyoxyethylene-polyoxypropylene block polymers
Silicones		
Taurates		

7.7.1.3 Antimicrobial Preservatives

Commonly used preservatives include Methyl hydroxyl benzoate, Propyl-hydroxybenzoate, Chlorocresol, Benzoic acid, Phenyl mercuric nitrate, benzalkonium chloride, Chlorhexidine acetate, benzyl alcohol and mercurial.

7.7.1.4 Antioxidants

These are powerful reducing agents, incorporated in to the formulation to prevent active ingredient from oxidation. Further these are classified based on its solubility viz. oil soluble and water soluble antioxidants.

Example: Butylated hydroxy anisole, Butylated hydroxy toluene, tocopherol etc.

7.7.1.5 Humectants

These are added to prevent semisolid preparation from drying out.

Example: Poly Ethylene Glycol, Glycerol or Sorbitol.

7.7.1.6 Flavouring Agents

Most commonly used flavouring agents are Lavender oil, Rose oil, Lemon oil, Almond oil.

7.7.1.7 Permeation Enhancers

Skin can act as a barrier and prevent deep penetration of drug molecules. With the introduction of various penetration enhancers, however, systemic drug delivery through the transdermal route has gained major footing. In addition to the use of penetration enhancers alone, their combination with co solvents that deliver a drug in solubilized form has led to the achievement of higher drug permeability

Examples: $DMSO_4$, surfactants, Menthol, Dimetyl acetamide, linalool, Lecithin, Limonene, Propylene glycol etc.

Penetration enhancer works by:

(a) Reversibly disordering the lamellar packing of stratum corneum
(b) Increasing the thermodynamic activity of the drug
(c) Solvent action
(d) Carrier mechanism of ionizable drugs
(e) Hydration of stratum corneum

7.7.1.8 Types of Gelling Agents

These are organic hydrocolloids or hydrophilic inorganic substances. Commonly used gelling agents are carbomer, sodium carboxymethyl cellulose, guar gum, methyl cellulose, locust bean gum, sodium alginate.

7.8 Preparation of Semisolids

Semisolids are prepared by either incorporating the active ingredient(s) into the chosen base or by melting the base and active ingredient(s) together.

A. *Incorporation method*: Ointment is prepared using mortar and pestle or on an ointment slab and spatula.

The active ingredient and the ointment base are mixed together until a uniform preparation is obtained. Before the incorporation of the active ingredient, it is often desirable to reduce the particle size of powder so the final product will not be gritty. Alternatively, solids may first be dissolved in small amount of a solvent (e.g., water or alcohol) and the solution is then mixed with the ointment base. This is called levigation. Alcoholic solutions of small volume may be added easily to both oleaginous or emulsion bases. Then continue this routine of mixing equal amounts of paste and base until the entire base has been added and you have a uniform preparation with a very small particle size. A mortar and pestle should be used for incorporating liquids into a base or for preparing larger quantities of an ointment.

B. *Fusion method***:** The fusion method is particularly useful when solid waxes are included in the ointment to add viscosity. In this method, first melt the substance with the highest melting point by using a water bath, but use as little heat as necessary. Then add the other ingredients on the basis of their decreasing melting points. When the entire mixture is liquefied, remove it from the water bath. Then stir the mixture until it congeals, to prevent possible separation and crystallization.

C. *By chemical reactions***:** In chemical method a new product is formed by chemical reaction, which involves both fusion and mechanical mixing. Best example of such method is Iodine ointment.

7.9   Semi Solid Preparation in Ophthalmic Drug Delivery

The eye is a unique organ from anatomical and physiological point of view, in that it contains several highly different structures with specific physiological functions. Ocular disposition and elimination of a therapeutic agent is dependent upon its physicochemical properties as well as the relevant ocular anatomy and physiology. The poor accessibility of a number of ocular regions to systemic circulation makes local delivery via topical administration the preferred route for the treatment of ocular diseases.

In ocular drug delivery, many physiological constraints prevent a successful drug delivery to the eye due to its protective mechanisms.

- The permeability barriers posed by cornea and other regions
- Tear washout and blinking reflexes
- Nasolachrymal drainage, lachrimation and tear dilution
- Less capacity of cul de sac (up to 7.5 μL)

Ophthalmic preparations, including solutions, suspensions, and ointments, can be applied topically to the cornea or instilled in the space between the eyeball and lower eyelid (the cul-de-sac or conjunctival sac of the lower lid.

7.9.1 Classification of Ocular Drug Delivery Systems

These can be classified on the basis of their physical forms as follows:

1. *Liquids*: Solutions, Suspensions, Sol to gel systems and Sprays.
2. *Solids*: Ocular inserts, Contact lenses, corneal shield.
3. *Semi-solids*: Ointments, Gels. Major advantage of selecting semisolid dosage form in an ophthalmic preparation is to increase the time of contact with the surface of the eye without washing away of the drug quickly due to tears.
4. *Miscellaneous*: Ocular iontophoresis, Vesicular systems, Mucoadhesive system.

Use of Hyaluronic acid, Use of Hydroxy Beta Cyclodextrin Ophthalmic dosage forms must meet the requirements of Sterility Tests.

7.10 Nasal Drug Delivery System

Nasal drug administration has been routinely used for administration of drugs for the upper respiratory tract and is now also being used as a viable alternative for the delivery of many systemic therapeutic agents. A number of dosage forms are common and include solutions, suspensions and gels ointments, sprays etc.

Nasal gels are semisolid preparations prepared for nasal application and can be for either local or systemic use, in a water soluble or water miscible vehicle where as Nasal ointments are prepared from either water miscible/soluble or oleaginous bases.

Advantages

- Lower doses,
- Rapid local therapeutic effect,
- Rapid systemic therapeutic blood levels,
- rapid onset of pharmacological activity, and
- Few side effects.
- Ideal for those drugs that undergo extensive hepatic first-pass elimination, gut wall metabolism, or destruction in GI fluids

Disadvantages

- The risk of patient-to-patient contamination is very high
- Non conventional route of application.

7.10.1   Formulation Aspect

Nasal and ophthalmic preparations contain a number of excipients, including vehicles, buffers, preservatives, tonicity adjusting agents, gelling agents and possibly antioxidants. Important in the formulation process is the use of ingredients that are nonirritating and compatible with the nose.

The requirements of a vehicle for nasal semisolids include:

1. *pH*: Generally, in the range of 5.5-7.5.
2. Mild buffer capacity.
3. *Isotonicity*: hyper tonicity may slow or even stop the nasal ciliary movement. Nasal fluid is isotonic with 0.9% sodium chloride solution.

   Examples: 0.9% sodium chloride, 1.7 % boric acid and 5.2% dextrose.
4. *Mucus viscosity*: A strongly hypertonic product may result in a slight drying effect and thickening of the mucous and hypotonic product affect on the efficiency of the cilia in mucous and particulate removal.
5. *Compatibility* with active ingredient.
6. *Stability*: Stability is largely influenced by pH, temperature, light, oxidation and other factors.
7. *Sterility*: Nasal preparations should be sterile.

7.10.2   Packing Storage and Labeling

Nasal preparations should be stored at either room or refrigerated temperatures and should not be frozen.

7.11 Rectal Drug Delivery

It is used for the symptomatic relief against anal and perianal pruritus, pain and inflammation associated with hemorrhoids, anal fissure, fistulas and proctitis. Rectal ointment should be applied several times in a day according to the severity of the condition. For intra-rectal use, apply the ointment with the help of special applicator.

Rectal tissues are much thicker than other gastro intestinal epithelial tissue. Bioavailability of this route depends upon pH of environment, lipid solubility of drug.

Rectal preparation includes ointments, creams, gels that are used for application to perianal area. Perianal area is the skin immediately surrounding anus. Substance applied rectally can be absorbed by diffusion into circulation via network of three hemorrhoid arteries (superior inferior and middle hemorrhoid artery)

Previously this route was used for bowel evacuation. But now a day's rectal route is widely use for administration of drugs like paracetamol, aspirin, indomethacin, theophyllin, barbiturates, chlorpromazine and several other anticonvulsant agents

7.11.1 Advantages, Applications and Uses

Several advantages of using rectal semisolids are:

1. Large surface area
2. The ability to bypass first-pass liver metabolism,
3. Prolongs the residence time and
4. Permeability to large molecular weight drugs, such as peptides and proteins. (insulin gels administered deep rectally)

Rectal preparations are used to treat anorectal pruritis, inflammation (hydrocortisone), discomfort with hemorrhoids (hydrocortisone), pain (pramoxine hydrochloride) Astringent (for example ZnO), protectants and lubricants (coca-butter, lanolin).

Risks of rectal semisolids are less frequent with rectal administration of drug including skin rash, dizziness, pain, headache, abdominal pain, nervousness, diarrhea, feeling unsteady or clumsy, and wheezing

Formulation of Rectal semisolids: Bases for preparation of anorectal ointment and creams are polyethylene glycol 300-3350, emulsion cream bases containing cetyl alcohol, cetyl ester wax, white petrolatum and mineral oil.

7.12 Vaginal Drug Delivery

The vagina has been explored as a favorable site for the local and systemic delivery of drugs used for the treatment of female-specific conditions. Vaginal delivery can be used for systemic as well as local action. The volume, viscosity and pH of vaginal fluid have a considerable influence on vaginal drug absorption. Drug permeation across the vaginal epithelium is via two main routes para cellular (between adjacent epithelial cells) and transcellular (across epithelial cells), which can occur by either passive diffusion, carrier mediated transport or endocytic processes. Several formulations are available for intravaginal therapy such as; tablets, hard and soft gelatin capsules, creams, suppositories, pessaries, foams, ointments, gels, films, tampons, vaginal rings, and douches.

Use of ointments, gels, or creams for vaginal applications provides high patient compliance, increased contact time for better release and absorption of the drug and also is less irritant when compared to other dosage forms.

Advantages

1. Avoid first pass effect
2. Accessibility and large surface area
3. Self and even single administration
4. Vaginal administration permits use of prolonged dosing, with continuous release of medicaments, and hence, longer interval between doses, improving user compliance
5. Vaginal epithelium has a lower enzyme activity compared to the GI tract
6. Permeability to large molecular weight drugs, such as peptides and proteins.

Disadvantages

1. The small volume of vaginal fluid makes dissolution a rate limiting step for systemic absorption of drugs from vaginal formulations
2. Cultural sensitivity
3. Personal hygiene
4. Gender specificity.

7.13 Quality Control Parameters

Due to the use of number of additives, it is necessary to evaluate the effectiveness of semisolid formulations. The various quality control parameters for semisolids are as follows:

7.13.1 pH

When applicable, semisolid drug products should be tested for pH at the time of batch release and designated stability test time points for batch-to-batch monitoring. Because most semisolid dosage forms contain very limited quantities of water or aqueous phase, pH measurements may be warranted only as a quality control measure, as appropriate.

7.13.2 Particle Size

Particle size of the active drug substance in semisolid dosage forms is determined and controlled at the formulation development stage. When applicable, semisolid drug products should be tested. For any change in the particle size or habit of the active drug substance at the time of batch release and designated stability test time points (for batch-to-batch monitoring) that could compromise the integrity and/or performance of the drug product, as appropriate.

7.13.3 *In-vitro* Drug Release

Flow thorough cell and Franz diffusion cell are used to measure drug release from semisolid dosage forms.

7.13.4 Viscosity Measurement

It is done with the help of Brook-field viscometer, Cone and plate viscometer and Penetrometer for consistency measurement.

7.13.5 Texture Analysis

Texture analyzer is used to detect:

(a) Flow characteristic

(b) Consistency

(c) Gel strength

7.13.6   Irritancy Test

Patch test: In this test 24 human volunteers are selected. Definite quantity of semisolid preparation is applied under occlusion daily on the back or volar forearm for 21 days. No visible reaction or erythema or edema or vesicular erosion should occur. A good ointment base shows no visible reaction.

Draize skin irritation test: A known amount of test substance is introduced under a one square inch gauge patch, the patch is applied to skin of 12 albino rabbits, (6 with intact skin) and (6 with abraded skin). After 24 hours the patches are removed and resulting reaction is evaluated for erythema and edema formation.

7.14 Storage and Packaging of Semisolids

Topical semisolid products are packed in either jar or tubes, whereas ophthalmic, nasal, vaginal and rectal semisolid products are almost always packed in tubes.   Ointment, creams and gels are most frequently packed in 5, 15 and 30 gm tubes. Ophthalmic ointments typically are packed in small aluminum or collapsible plastic tubes holding 3-5 gm of ointment.

The semisolid preparation should maintain its pharmaceutical integrity throughout shelf-life when stored at the temperature indicated on the label. Special storage recommendations or limitations are indicated in individual monographs. Storage of semisolids should be at temperatures not exceeding 25° unless otherwise authorized. They should not be allowed to freeze and must be stored in a well-closed container. The containers are preferably collapsible metal tubes from which the preparation may be readily extruded. If the preparation is sterile, store in a sterile, airtight, tamper-proof container.

7.15 Advancement in Semisolid Dosage Form

Advancement in semisolid dosage form allows modified release as well as flexibility in route of administration. Novel creams now a days are provided with nanoparticles and microspheres, which has an excellent emollient effect, with better spread ability, and less staining than oleaginous ointments.

7.15.1   Creams

Creams containing microspheres: Microsphere acts as a reservoir releasing an active ingredient over an extended period of time maintaining effective drug concentration in the skin and at the same time, reducing undesired side effects

Lamellar faced creams: Lamellar Cream is a highly advanced, multi use, soft cream with lamellar structure. This has advantages of easy application, fast absorption and leaves no residue on the skin.

Cream containing lipid nanoparticles: Solid lipid nanoparticles possess the advantages of better drug penetration because of small particle size and higher amount of drug encapsulation. Occlusive properties on the skin can be obtained as a continuous film forms when the gel or cream is applied.

7.15.2   Gels

- Controlled release gels
- Organogels

Organogels have long been tried as a matrix for transdermal delivery systems because of its ability to improve the transport rate of the bioactive agents, longer shelf life, ease of preparation and thermo-reversible nature.

- Extended release gels
- Bio adhesive gels
- Thermo-reversible gels
- Thermo-sensitive *in situ* Hydro gels
- pH responsive complexation gel

These are the aqueous polymeric solutions which undergo reversible sol to gel transformation under the influence of environmental conditions like temperature and pH which results in *in-situ* hydrogel formation

Applications

- Helps to deliver labile bio macromolecule such as proteins and genes.
- Immobilization of cells

- Tissue engineering
- Controlled release drug delivery

Novel advances in semisolid applications: There are various advancements in delivery of drugs (Gels, jellies, ointments, creams) in ocular, topical, vaginal, rectal routes.

Delivery of monoclonal antibody using semisolid dosage form. Several novel drug delivery systems like liposomes, niosomes, microemulsions, nanoparticles, micelles and microspheres were explored for topical therapy.

- Topical delivery of vitamin A.

- **Liposomal transdermal delivery:** Recently, Liposome's have shown great potential as novel drug carriers for dermal and transdermal systems. One of the advantages of using liposomes as transdermal drug carriers is that both lipophilic as well as hydrophilic drugs can be incorporated and also, serve as a reservoir for the prolonged release of drugs beneath various skin layers. Because they are nongreasy and nontacky, liposomal semisolid preparations are also cosmetically acceptable.

8 Parenteral Products

8.1 Introduction

Parenteral preparations are sterile preparations intended for the administration by injections, infusions or implantation into the animal or human body. The term parenteral literally means 'Para and Enteron' i.e., to avoid the gut (gastrointestinal tract). Thus, parenterals are injectable drugs enter the body directly and are not required to be absorbed in the gastrointestinal tract before they show their effect. Parenteral routes of administration usually have a more rapid onset of action (show their effects more quickly) than other routes of administration. Parenteral products must be sterile. The parenteral route of administration does have its disadvantages like it hurts, it is not a convenient route, and once administered the injected drug cannot be retrieved.

8.1.1 Advantages of Parenterals

- Quick onset of action
- It provides immediate therapeutic action (Emergency condition)
- Accurate dosing
- Suitable for non-cooperative and unconscious patient, who cannot take oral medication
- It minimizes the first pass effect
- It provides more bioavailability
- Prolonged duration of action.

8.1.2 Disadvantages of Parenterals

- It should be administered aseptically
- Only trained personnel are required to administer
- It induces pain at the site of injection
- Risk of infection of some emboli

- Self administration is not possible
- Higher cost
- Difficulty in drug removal or reversal.

8.2   Route of Parenteral Administration

Routes of administration are generally classified by the location at which the substance is applied. The major routes of parenteral administration are intravenous, Intramuscular and subcutaneous as depicted in Figure 8.1 and Table 8.1.

8.2.1 Intravenous Route

Intravenous medication is injected directly into a vein either to obtain an extremely rapid and predictable response or to avoid irritation of other tissues. This route of administration also provides maximum availability and assurance in delivering the drug to the site of action. However, a major danger of this route of administration is that the rapidity of absorption. Large proximal veins, that are those located in the forearm, are most commonly used for IV administration.

8.2.2 Intramuscular Route

The intramuscular route is used when drugs are injected deeply into the striated muscle fibers that lie beneath the subcutaneous layer. The principal sites of injection are the gluteal (buttocks), deltoid (upper arm), and vastus lateralis (lateral thigh) muscles. The usual volumes injected range from 0.5 to 2.0 mL, with volumes up to 4.0 mL sometimes being given (in divided doses) in the gluteal or thigh areas. There are numerous dosage forms available for this route of administration: solutions, oil-in-water (o/w) or water in-oil (w/o) emulsions, suspensions (aqueous or oily base), colloidal suspensions, and reconstitutable powders. The major clinical problem arising from IM injections is muscle or neuron damage. This route provides a means of sustained release of drugs formulated as aqueous or oily solutions or suspensions.

8.2.3 Subcutaneous Route

This route involves the injection of the drug into the loose connective and adipose tissue beneath the dermis. Subcutaneous injections are usually administered in volumes up to 2 mL using a 1/2- to 1-in. 23-gauge needle. Drugs given by this route will have a slower onset of action than by the IM or IV routes, and total absorption may also be less. Heparin and insulin are among the drugs generally administered by subcutaneous route. Highly acidic or alkaline drugs causing irritation, pain, inflammation and/or necrosis of tissues cannot be administered by subcutaneous route.

8.2.4 Intrathecal Route

The intrathecal route involves the administration of a drug directly into the cerebrospinal fluid at any level of the cerebrospinal axis. This route is commonly used in cesarean operations to anesthetise pregnant women.

8.2.5 Intraarterial Route

The intraarterial route involves injecting a drug directly into an artery. This technique is not simple and may require a surgical procedure to reach the artery. This route is used to administer radiopaque contrast media for viewing an organ, such as the heart or kidney. This route is generally used for organ specific chemotherapy.

8.2.6 Intradermal Route

In this route, the drug is injected into the skin layers. Ideally, the drug is placed within the dermis. The intradermal route is used almost exclusively for diagnostic purpose. Volumes are normally given at 0.05 mL/dose, and the solutions are isotonic.

8.2.7 Intracisternal Route

The intra-cisternal route involves administration of a drug directly into caudal region of brain between cerebellum and medulla oblongata. This route is mainly used for diagnostic purpose. It could be performed by direct injection into the cisterna magna.

8.2.8 Intraperitoneal Route

The route of administration in which the injection or infusion is given directly into the peritoneal cavity or directly into an abdominal organ, such as the kidney, liver or bladder is known as intraperitoneal route. This route is mostly employed to dialyze and remove different toxic substances from the body.

8.2.9 Intrapleural Route

Injection given into the pleural cavity is called as intrapleural route. This route may be used for irrigation purposes or for repeated injections of drugs.

8.2.10   Intraarticular

Injection given into a joint space. It is used in treating osteoarthritis.

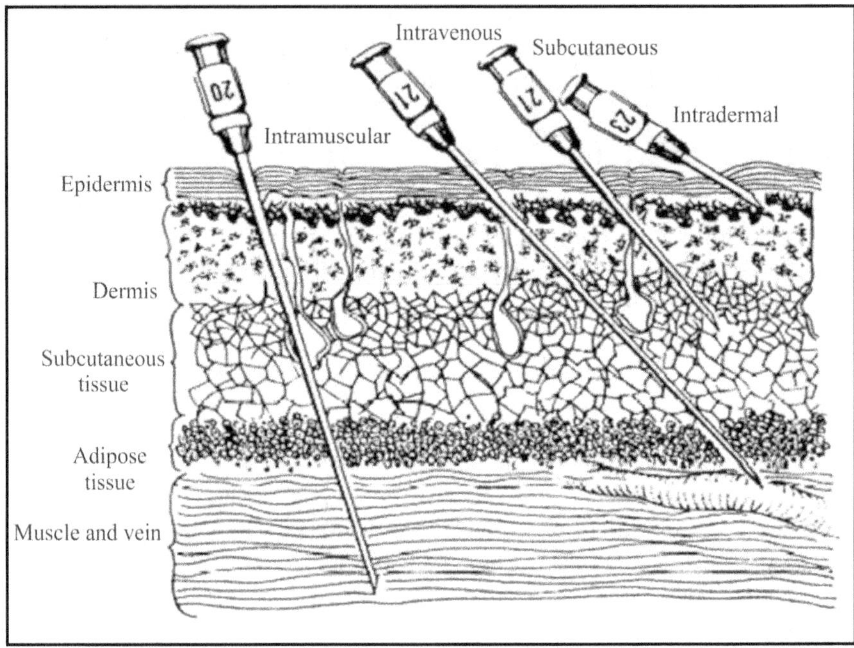

FIGURE 8.1 Routes of parenterals administration.

TABLE 8.1

Routes of parenterals administration

Route	Injection site
Intravenous Route	vein
Intramuscular Route	Muscle tissue
Subcutaneous Route	Subcutaneous tissue of skin
Intrathecal Route	Subarachnoid space of spinal cord
Intra-arterial Route	Artery
Intradermal Route	Dermis of skin

Table 8.1 *contd...*

Route	Injection site
Intra cisternal Route	caudal region of brain
Intraperitoneal route	Peritoneal cavity
Intrapleural route	pleural cavity
Intra articular	joint space

8.4 Types of Parenteral Formulation

- Injections,
- Infusions,
- Concentrates for injections or infusions,
- Powders for injections or infusions,
- Gels for injections,
- Implants.

8.4.1 Large Volume Parenteral (LVP) Solutions

LVP solutions are typically bags or bottles containing larger volumes of intravenous solutions. Common uses of LVP solutions without additives include, correction of electrolyte and fluid balance disturbances, nutrition, as a vehicle for administering other drugs. Large volume parenteral solutions are packaged in containers holding 100mL or more. Preservatives are not used in LVP's as the amount needed to preserve them would be large and if the same amount of preservatives be injected into the patients would be harmful.

8.4.2 Small Volume Parenteral (SVP) Solutions

Small volume parenteral (SVP) solutions are usually 100 mL or less and are packaged depending on the intended use. SVPs are typically packed as ampoules, vials, small bags and prefilled syringes. The detail of specification of both SVP and LVP is shown in Table 8.2.

TABLE 8.2

Comparison of SVP and LVP

	SVP	**LVP**
Packing	100 mL or less	100-1000 mL
Route	IV/IM/SC	Mostly IV
Preservative	Used	Not necessary
Form	Solution/suspension/ emulsion	Mostly solution
Use	Therapeutic agent/ Diagnostic	Replacement/Nutritional, Detoxification

8.4.3 Specialized Large Volume Parenterals

Large volume Parenterals conventionally considered as saline only, but Parenterals has a wide range of specialized LVPs as:

8.4.3.1 Hyper Alimentation Solutions

Parenteral hyper alimentation involves administration of large amounts of nutrients (*e.g.*, carbohydrates, amino acids, lipids, and vitamins) to a patient who is unable to take food orally for several weeks

8.4.3.2 Cardioplegia Solutions

Cardioplegia solutions are large-volume parenteral solutions used in heart surgery to help prevent ischemic injury to the myocardium during the time the blood supply to the heart is clamped off and during reperfusion, as well as to maintain a bloodless operating field and to make the myocardium flaccid.

8.4.3.3 Peritoneal Dialysis Solutions

The sterile peritoneal dialysis solutions are infused continuously into the abdominal cavity, bathing the peritoneum, and are then continuously withdrawn. The purpose of peritoneal dialysis is to remove toxic substances from the body or to aid and accelerate the excretion function normal to the kidneys.

8.4.3.4 Irrigating Solutions

Irrigating solutions are intended to irrigate, flush and aid in cleansing body cavities and wounds.

8.5 Formulation Aspects

Parenteral formulations circumvent the skin and directly introduce in to the systemic circulation therefore, must be free from contamination, pyrogen free, sterile and safe. Special Considerations requires for the formulation of parenteral preparation and typically requires specific considerations on the type and quality of excipients used.

8.5.1 Criteria for Parenterals

- Sterility
- Stability
- Pyrogen
- Isotonicity
- pH

pH Considerations: A parenteral product should be formulated with a pH close to physiological pH. Often, the pH selected for the product is a compromise between the pH of maximum stability, solubility and physiological acceptability. The first step in selecting a suitable formulation pH will be the generation of pH/ stability and pH/solubility profiles.

This type of information is often available in the preformulation data. The target pH for maximum physiological acceptability is approximately pH 7.4. In practice, however, a reasonably wide pH range can be tolerated, particularly when dosing is via the IV route, and dilution with blood is rapid. In these circumstances pHs ranging from 2 to 12 can be tolerated. The dilution rate is slower when administration is via the intramuscular route and decreases further when the subcutaneous route is used. For this reason, pH ranges of 3 to 11 and 3 to 6, respectively, are recommended for these routes

A pH outside 3-9 range should be avoided if possible, since a pH of greater than 9 can cause tissue necrosis, whereas a pH of less than 3 may cause pain. The buffers most commonly encountered in parenteral products are phosphate, citrate or acetate. Phosphate is useful for buffering around physiological pH, whereas acetate and citrate are used when the required pH is lower. Buffers which are encountered in parenteral products are Acetate, Ammonium, Ascorbate, Benzoate, Bicarbonate, Citrate, Lactate and Tartrate salt.

Tonicity considerations: Parenteral products should be isotonic (between 280 and 290 mOsm/L). Osmolarity is the number of milliosmoles/liter (mOsm/L) of solution. Hypertonic solutions are preferable to hypotonic solutions because of the risk of haemolysis associated with the latter. Mannitol, dextrose or other inert excipients can also be used and may be preferable if the addition of sodium chloride is likely to have an adverse effect on the formulation. Tonicity modifiers have dual functionality as mannitol often functions both to increase the osmolarity and to act as a bulking agent in lyophilized formulations.

8.5.2 Vehicles

Parenteral drugs are formulated as solutions, suspensions, emulsions and powders to be reconstituted as solutions. This section describes the components such as, Vehicles and additives commonly used in parenteral formulations.

8.5.2.1 Aqueous Vehicles

Water for injection (WFI) is the most widely used solvent for parenteral preparations.

There are many different grades of water used for pharmaceutical purposes. Several are described in USP monographs that specify uses, acceptable methods of preparation, and quality attributes. These waters can be divided into two general types: bulk waters, which are typically produced on site where they are used; and packaged waters, which are produced, packaged, and sterilized to preserve microbial quality throughout their packaged shelf life. There are several specialized types of packaged waters, differing in their designated applications, packaging limitations, and other quality attributes. For the parenteral products, the most usual vehicle is water. Water is most abundantly available, cheap, safe, non-toxic and non-irritating. Water is widely used as a raw material, ingredient, and solvent in the processing, formulation, and manufacture of parenteral products.

- ***Water for injection, USP*:** Water for Injection USP is chemically designated water and is used as an excipient in the production of parenteral and other preparations where product endotoxin content must be controlled, and in other pharmaceutical applications, such as cleaning of certain equipment and parenteral product-contact components. Water for injection must be designed to minimize or prevent microbial contamination as well as remove incoming endotoxin from the starting water.

- ***Sterile water for injection, USP***: Sterile water for injection, USP is a sterile, nonpyrogenic, solute-free preparation of distilled water for injection. It is for use only as a sterile solvent or diluent vehicle for drugs or solutions suitable for parenteral administration. The pH is 5.5 (5.0 to 7.0). It contains no bacteriostatic, antimicrobial agent or added buffer and is intended only for single-dose injection after admixture with an appropriate solute or solution and must be made approximately isotonic prior to use.

- ***Purified water***: Purified water is used as excipient in the production of nonparenteral preparations and in other pharmaceutical applications, such as cleaning of certain equipment and nonparenteral product-contact components. It is also to be used for all tests and assays. Purified water must meet the requirements for ionic and organic chemical purity and must be protected from microbial contamination.

- ***Bacteriostatic water for injection***: Bacteriostatic water for injection is sterile Water for Injection to which one or more suitable antimicrobial preservatives have been added. It is intended to be used as a diluent in the preparation of parenteral products, most typically for multi-dose products that require repeated content withdrawals. It may be packaged in single-dose or multiple-dose containers not larger than 30mL.

- ***Sterile water for irrigation***: Sterile Water for Irrigation is a sterile, hypotonic, nonpyrogenic irrigating fluid or pharmaceutic aid entirely composed of Sterile Water for Injection packaged and sterilized in single-dose containers of larger than 1 L in size. It is utilized for a variety of clinical indications, because of its low refractive index (1.3325), water provides excellent visibility during endoscopic urological procedures. It is also utilized as a pharmaceutic aid for sterile irrigation, washing, rinsing and dilution purposes.

8.5.2.2 Nonaqueous Vehicles

A nonaqueous solvent or a mixed aqueous/nonaqueous solvent system may be necessary to stabilize drug.

Oily: A major class of nonaqueous solvents are the fixed oils. The most commonly used oils are corn oil, cottonseed oil, peanut oil, and sesame oil.

8.5.3 Antioxidants

Salts of sulfur dioxide, including bisulfite, metasulfite and a metal chelator, such as disodium EDTA are the most common antioxidants used in aqueous parenterals, or an antioxidant compound, such as ascorbic acid or sodium metabisulphite, may be considered.

8.5.4 Antimicrobial Agents

A suitable preservative system is required in all multiple dose parenteral products to inhibit the growth of microorganisms accidentally introduced during withdrawal of individual doses. The minimum concentration of preservative should be used, which gives the required level of efficacy. The most commonly used preservatives and their typical concentrations are as shown in Table 8.3.

TABLE 8.3

Preservatives and their typical concentrations

Sr. No.	Preservatives	Typical concentration (%)
1	Benzyl alcohol	1–2
2	Chlorbutanol	0.5
3	Methylparaben	0.1–0.18
4	Propylparaben	0.01–0.02
5	Phenol	0.2–0.5
6	Thiomersal	0.01

8.5.5 Buffers

Many drugs require a certain pH range to maintain product stability. Buffer systems for parenterals consist of either a weak base and the salt of a weak base or a weak acid and the salt of a weak acid. Buffer systems commonly used for injectable products are acetates, citrates, and phosphates as shown in Table 8.4.

TABLE 8.4

Buffers use in parenterals

Buffer	pH Range
Acetate	3.8-5.8
Ammonium	8.25-10.25
Ascorbate	3.0-5.0

Table 8.4 *contd....*

Buffer	pH Range
Benzoate	6.0-7.0
Bicarbonate	4.0-11.0
Citrate	2.1-6.2
Glycine	8.8-10.8
Phosphate	3.0-8.0
Tartrate	2.0-5.3

8.5.6 Solubilizing Agents/Co-solvents

Commonly used co solvents for parenteral products are glycerin, ethanol, propylene glycol, polyethylene glycol and N, N-dimethylacetamide. Generally, the polysorbates, are frequently encountered in parenteral products at very low levels (0.05 percent).

8.5.7 Tonicity Adjustment Agents

It is important that injectable solutions that are to be given intravenously are isotonic, or nearly so. Dextrose, sodium chloride, or potassium chloride are commonly used to achieve isotonicity in a parenteral formula.

8.5.8 Protectants

These are the materials capable of protecting the substance from lyophilisation process. A protectant is a substance that is added to a formulation to protect against loss of activity caused by some stress that is introduced by the manufacturing process or to prevent loss of active ingredients by adsorption to process equipment or to primary packaging materials.

Protectants are used primarily in protein formulations, liposomal formulations, and vaccines. For example, cryoprotectants and lyoprotectants are used to inhibit loss of integrity of the active substance resulting from freezing and drying, respectively. Polyethylene glycol protects lactate dehydrogenase and phosphofructokinase from damage by freezing, but does not protect either protein from damage by freeze-drying. Compounds such as sucrose and trehalose are effective lyoprotectants for both proteins

Another type of protectant is used to prevent loss of active substance usually a protein and usually present at a very low concentration by adsorption to materials or equipment in the manufacturing process or to components of the primary package. Human serum albumin (HSA) may be used as a protectant against adsorptive loss of proteins present at low concentrations.

E.g.: Sugars-sucrose,

Trehalose Aminoacid-glycine,

Lysine Polymers-dextran,

Poly ethylene glycol

8.6   General Manufacturing Process

The production facility and its associated equipment must be designed, constructed, and operated properly for the manufacture of a sterile product to be achieved at the quality level required for safety and effectiveness. The overall Manufacturing process of Parenterals are shown in Figure 8.2.

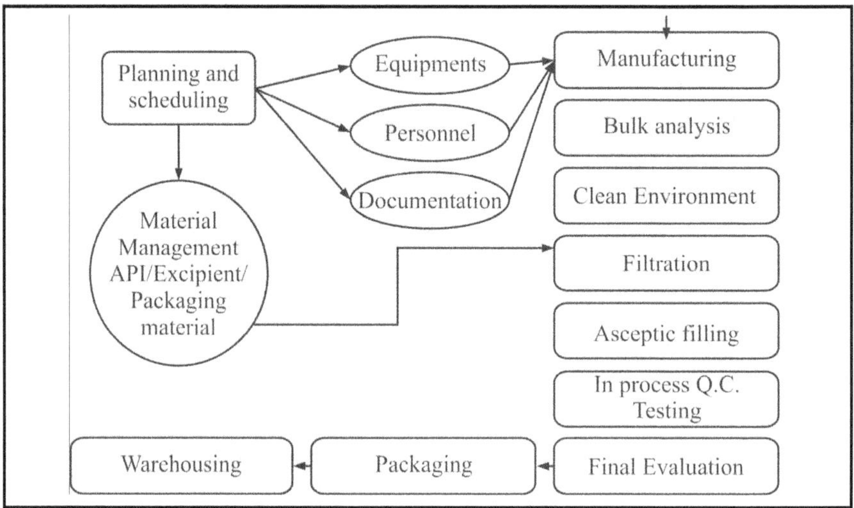

FIGURE 8.2 Manufacturing process of parenterals.

Production Facilities: In manufacturing of parenterals, control of contamination and cross contamination plays important role by design consideration.

The chart for ideal process flow of material is as shown in Figure 8.3.

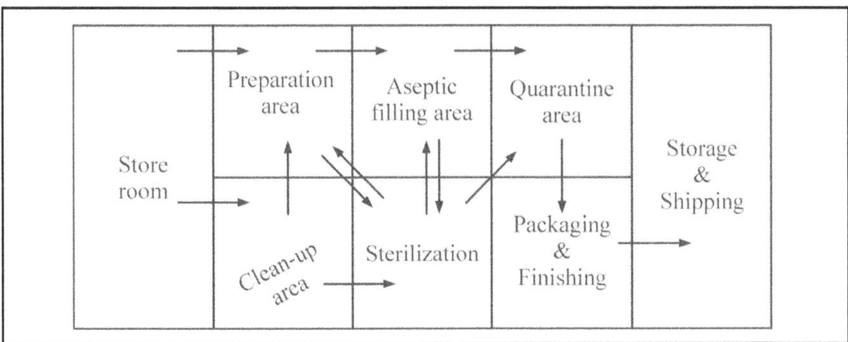

FIGURE 8.3 Process flow of material.

Manufacturing operations are divided into two categories; firstly, those where the product is terminally sterilised, and secondly those which are conducted aseptically at some or all stages.

Types of sterile products processing:

1. ***Terminally Sterilised*:** usually involves filling and sealing product containers under high-quality environmental conditions

2. ***Sterilized by filtration*:** Filters having nominal pore size 0.22 µm or less are used for filtration

3. ***Aseptic preparations*:** In an aseptic sterlisation, the drug product, container, and closure are sterilized separately and then brought together.

Facility Design

- Manufacturing areas designed for aseptic processing should be smooth easily cleaned surfaces.

- Designed to control the manufacturing environment (personnel and process).

- Adequate and separate areas, for various activities (testing, manufacturing).

- HEPA-filtered air in manufacturing areas.

- Material and personnel flows designed to maximize efficiency and minimize product mix-ups and concurrent not complete.

Functional Areas

To achieve the goal of a manufactured sterile product of exceptionally high quality, many functional production areas are involved:

- Warehousing or procurement
- Compounding (formulation)
- Filtration
- Aseptic filling
- Packaging, labelling, and quarantine.

The design and control of an aseptic area is directed toward reducing the presence of contaminants (dust, fibers etc).

Classification of Clean Rooms

Due to the extremely high standards of cleanliness and purity that must be met by parenteral products, it has become standard practice to prescribe specifications for the environments (clean rooms) in which these products are manufactured. The class is directly related to the number of particles per cubic foot of air equal to or greater than 0.5 micron.

- *Class* **100,000:** Particle count not to exceed a total of 100,000 particles per cubic foot of a size 0.5μ and larger
- *Class* **10,000:** Particle count not to exceed a total or 10,000 particles per cubic foot of a size 0.5μ and larger
- *Class* **1,000:** Particles count not to exceed a total of 1000 particles per cubic foot of a size 0.5μ and larger
- *Class* **100:** Particles count not to exceed a total of 100 particles per cubic foot of a size 0.5μ and larger

The various operations of component preparation, product preparation, filling and sterilization should be carried out in separate areas within a clean area. These areas are classified into four grades as shown in Table 8.5

Grade **A:** The local zone for high risk operations, *e.g.*: filling zone, Ampoule sealing etc. Such conditions are provided by a laminar air flow work station.

Grade **B:** Used for aseptic preparation and filling,

Grade **C** *and* **D:** Clean areas for carrying out less critical stages in the manufacture of sterile products.

TABLE 8.5

Various grades of clean area

Grade	Maximum number of particle grade permitted per m³		Maximum number of viable micro-organism per m³
	0.5 – 5 µm	> 5 µm	
A	3 500	None	Less than 1
B	3 500	None	5
C	3 50000	2000	100
D	3 500000	20000	500

Clean area zones as per gazette of India (Figure 8.4)

- *White zone*: Grade A (high risk operations such as aseptic filling)

- *Grey zone*: Grade B and C (Moderate risk operation such as aseptic preparation and filtration)

- *Black zone*: Grade D (represent less critical area used for Packaging and storage)

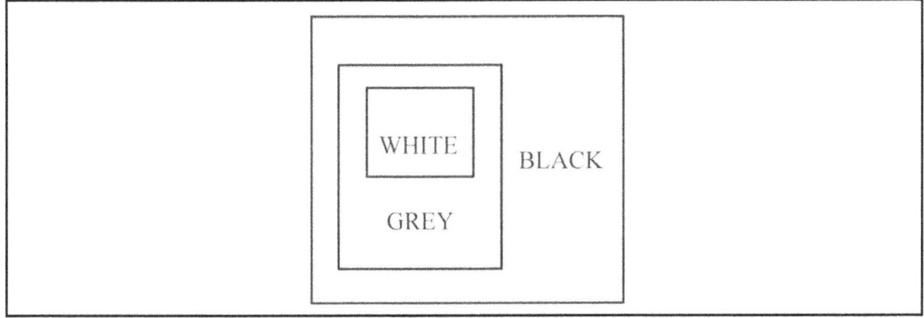

FIGURE 8.4 Clean area zones as per gazzete of India.

Air Cleaning: Since air is one of the greatest potential sources of contaminants in clean rooms, special attention must be given to air drawn into clean rooms by the heating, ventilating, and air conditioning (HVAC) systems. The manufacture of sterile products should be carried out in clean areas, entry to which should be through airlocks for personnel and/or for equipment and materials. Clean areas should be maintained to an appropriate cleanliness standard and supplied with air which has passed through filters of an appropriate efficiency.

Personnel Flow: The movement of personnel should be planned and minimized during the design of individual plant areas. Each individual production area should have a smooth and efficient personnel flow pattern, rather than a discontinuous or crowded pattern, which may increase the chances of contamination of product.

8.7 Pyrogens

8.7.1 Nature and Source

Pyrogens are the metabolic products of bacteria. Chemically, they are lipid substances associated with a carrier molecule, which is usually a polysaccharide. The carrier may also be a peptide. These carriers increase the solubility of the lipid. Pyrogens are produced by many microorganisms including bacteria, yeasts and moulds. Most potent pyrogens are the endotoxins produced from the cell walls of the Gram-negative bacteria. When pyrogens are introduced into a body they produce a mark response of fever with body ache and vasoconstriction within an onset of 1 hour. These products are not destroyed by autoclaving, hence must be prevented from getting into water. So the water being taken for parenteral preparation must be apyrogenic.

Pyrogens are fever producing substances, which are metabolic products of microorganisms. It enters the bloodstream and binds to Lipopolysaccharide Binding Protein (LPB). LPB takes it to the reticuloendothelial system (RES). The receptor cells in the RES are the circulating mononuclear cells. This attachment to the receptor cells causes the production of proinflammatory cytokines. These cytokines are interleukin-1 (IL-1), interleukin-6 (IL-6), and tumor necrosis factor-α (TNFα). These factors produce inflammation and fever. Pyrogens have a high molecular weight, often, more than 1,000,000.

The various sources of pyrogens by which parenteral formulation gets contaminated are drugs, vehicle, excipients, equipment, containers, environment and facilities used in manufacturing may be the sources of pyrogens. The method of storage in between preparation and sterilization also may cause the development of pyrogens. If unintentionally, pyrogens are injected into a patient, they may bring about the following physiological changes:

- Erythema at the injection site
- Pain in the legs and trunk
- General discomfort
- High temperature

Pyrogens, if present in large volume parenterals, can be especially dangerous, as they would be present in large quantities and are given intravenously

8.7.2 Elimination of Pyrogens

Pyrogens can be destroyed by:

- Heating at high temperatures. A typical procedure for depyrogenation of glassware and equipment is maintaining a dry heat temperature of 250 °C for 45 min. Exposure of 650 °C for 1 min or 180 °C for 4 hours, likewise, will destroy pyrogens.
- Heating with strong alkali, dilute acids or oxidizing solutions
- Reverse osmosis
- Distillation.
- Adsorption on adsorptive agents
- Ultrafiltration
- Anion-Exchange Resins and Positively Charged Membrane Filters

8.8 Quality Control Tests for Parenterals

The quality of parenterals is the sum of all parameters that contribute to safety, efficacy and therapeutic efficacy of the drug. Following are the tests for parenteral products.

1. Weight variation or content uniformity
2. Particulate matter in injections
3. Bacterial endotoxin test
4. Pyrogen test
5. Sterility test

8.8.1 Weight Variation or Content Uniformity Test

This test is intended for sterile solids used for parenteral preparation. The weight of 10 individual sterile units is noted and the content is removed from them and empty individual sterile unit is weighed again. Then net weight is calculated by subtracting empty sterile unit weight from gross weight.

The content of active ingredient in each sterile unit is calculated by performing the assay according to the individual monographs. The content in 10 sterile units is calculated by performing the assay. The dose uniformity is met if the amount of active ingredient is within the range of 85-115.0% of label claim as determine by the content uniformity method or weight variation method. The dose uniformity is also met if the potency value is 100% in the individual monograph or less of label claim multiplied by average of limits specified for potency in individual monograph divided by 100 provided that the relative standard deviation in both the cases is equal to or less than 6.0%. If one unit is outside the range of 85-115.0%, and none of the sterile unit is outside the range of 75-125.0% and if the relative standard deviation of the resultant is greater than 6.0% then, the fore mentioned test is carried for 20 more sterile units. The sterile units meet the requirements if not more than one unit is outside the range of 85-115%, no unit is outside the range of 75-125.0% and the calculated relative standard deviation is NMT 7.8%.

8.8.2 Particulate Matter in Injections

The preparations intended for parenteral use should be free from particulate matter and should be clear when inspected visually. Two methods are described by USP according to the filled volume of the product to be tested. For large volume parenterals (LVP's), a filtration followed by microscopic examination procedure is used. For small volume parenterals (SVP's) a light obscuration based sensor containing electronic liquid born we particle counter system is used.

The USP standards are met if the LVP's under test containing not more than 50 particles per ml of 10 μm, and not more than 5 particles per mL of 25 μm in an effective linear dimensional fashion. The USP standards are met if the SVP's under test contain no more than 10,000 particles per container of 10 μm, and not more than 1000 particles per container of 25 μm in an effective spherical diameter.

8.8.3 Pyrogen Test

Basically tests performed to detect the presence of pyrogens in sterile parenteral products are:

8.8.3.1 Rabbit Test

It is performed by using rabbits as test animals. Initially 10 mL/kg body weight of animal is injected through rabbit vein at 37 $\pm$ 2 °C within ten minutes from start of administration. The temperatures are recorded at 1, 2 and 3 hours after injection. The requirements of USP are met if the rise in temperature of individual rabbit is not more than 0.6 °C and the sum of rise in temperature of three rabbits is not more than 1.4 °C. If anyone rabbit shows a rise in temperature of more than 0.6 °C and sum of rise in temperature of three rabbits exceeds 1.4 °C then the test is repeated using 5 rabbits. The requirements are met if 3 out of 8 rabbits shows an individual rise in temperature of not more than 0.6 °C and sum of maximum rise in temperature of 8 rabbits is not more than 3.7 °C.

8.8.3.2 LAL Test

LAL (Limulus Amebocyte Lysate) test is used to characterize the bacterial endotoxin that may be present. The USP reference standard contains 10,000 USP endotoxins per vial. The LAL reagent is used for gel-clot formation. The test is performed using stated amounts of volumes of products, standard, positive control, negative control of endotoxin. The tubes are incubated at 37 ± 1 °C FOR 60 ± 2 min. When the tubes are inverted at 180 °C angle, formation of firm gel confirms positive reaction. While formation of a viscous gel that doesn't maintain its integrity or absence of a firm gel confirms negative reaction.

8.8.4 Sterility Test

Sterility is the most important and   absolutely essential   characteristic of parenteral   products.   The   methods   which   are   used   to perform sterility tests are

(A) Direct transfer method.

(B) Membrane filtration method.

Growth promotion medium and incubation conditions are selected based on the test microorganism according to USP and is listed in Table 8.6.

TABLE 8.6

USP sterility tests growth promotion microorganisms

Medium	Test microorganisms	Incubation	
		Temperature (^{0}C)	Conditions
Fluid thioglycollate	Bacillus subtillis	30 to 35	Aerobic
	Candida albicans	30 to 35	
	Bacteroides vulgates	30 to 35	
Alternative thioglycollate	Bacteroides vulgates	30 to 35	Anaerobic
Soybean-casein digest		20 to 25	Aerobic
	Candida albicans	20 to 25	

A. Direct Transfer Method: It is a traditional sterility test method in which direct aseptic transfer of specified volume from test container (Table 8.7) to culture medium and incubated for 14 days and visual observation of medium is done on 3rd, 4th, 5th, 7th, 8th and 14th day.

B. Membrane Filtration Method: Membrane filtration technique is suitable for liquids, soluble powders with bacteriostatic or fungi static properties, oils, creams and ointments. This method basically involves filtration of sample through membrane filters of porosity 0.22 micron and diameter 47 mm with flow rate of 55-75 mL of water per minute at a pressure of 70 mm of mercury. The filtration is assisted under vacuum, after filtration is completed the membrane is cut into 2 halves and one halve is placed in one or two test tubes containing medium.

Test meets the requirements when no growth is observed and if growth is observed then the test is repeated in the second stage and generally second stage is repeated with double the number of specimens tested in first stage, when the test was found to be conducted under faulty or inadequate aseptic techniques.

8.8   Packaging and Labelling of Parenterals

A thorough understanding of the regulatory guidance related to packaging components and the potential interaction between the drug and its primary packaging is critical when selecting the parenteral packaging system. By selecting the proper packaging components one can reduce the risk of loss caused when active ingredients, preservatives, stabilizers and buffer systems extract materials from the elastomer.

Any container for parenteral product should maintain the integrity of the product as a sterile, pyrogen free until it is used. It should also be attractive, allow the withdrawal of the contents and be strong enough to withstand processing and shipping; and importantly it should not interact with the product.

The packaging of parenteral products presents unique challenges in terms of the requirements for the packaging components to withstand sterilization prior to use and the requirement for the complete primary pack to maintain sterility throughout the shelf-life of the product. Primary packaging for parenterals can be either made of glass or polymer. Traditionally, SVPs have been packaged in ampoules which are heat sealed after filling. For products packaged in vials, a suitable rubber stopper must be selected. Glass seems to be the material of choice for containers for parenteral products. Glass containers may either be sealed or closed with rubber stoppers. Containers of Type I glass are best for aqueous preparations.

TABLE 8.7

Liquid quantities for USP sterility test

Container content (mL)	Minimum volume taken from each container for each medium	Medium use for direct transfer of volume from each container (mL)	Minimum volume of each	Number of containers per medium
			Used for membrane representing total volume from the appropriate number of containers	
Less than 10	1 mL or entire contents if less than 1 mL	15	100	20 (40 if each does not contain sufficient volume for both media)
10 to less than 50	5 mL	40	100	20
50 to less than 100	10 mL	80	100	20
50 to less than 100 intended for administration	Entire contents	-	100	10
100 to 500	Entire contents	-	100	10
>500	500 mL	-	100	10

Plastics used in the packaging of parenteral products are based on polyethylene or polypropylene.

Rubber is the material of choice for closures for multi-dose vials, intravenous fluid bottles. Rubber closures permit the introduction of a needle from a hypodermic syringe into a multi-dose vial and provide for resealing of the vial after the needle is withdrawn.

The label must state:

- The name of the preparation.
- The percentage content of drug of a liquid preparation,
- The amount of active ingredient of a dry preparation,
- The volume of liquid to be added to prepare an injection or suspension from a dry preparation,
- The route of administration.
- A statement of storage conditions.
- Date of expiry
- The label must indicate the name of the manufacturer and the Batch number

Preparations labelled for use as dialysis, hemofiltration, or irrigation solutions must meet the requirements for injections, other than those relating to volume, and must also bear on the label statements that they are not intended for intravenous injection. Injections intended for veterinary use are so labeled.

8.9   Recent Advancement in Parenteral Formulation

Novel approach for parenteral system provides drug release in controlled manner at a selected site without undesirable interactions at the other sites. This is achieved by two approaches. The first approach involves chemical modification of a parent compound to a derivative which is activated only at the targeted site. The second approach utilizes carriers such as liposomes, microspheres, nanoparticles and macromolecules to direct the drug to its site of action. Targeted and controlled drug release is an effective approach in avoidance of hepatic first pass metabolism, rapid onset of action, better patient compliance, enhancement of bioavailability.

Colloidal Dispersions

- Limosomes
- Niosomes
- Polymeric Micelles
- Nano suspension
- Nano Emulsion

- Solid Lipid Nano particles
- Released Erythrocytes

Implants: Implant represents novel approach in the use of solid dosage forms as parenteral product. Implants are insert under the skin by cutting and stitching it alter insertion of the sterile tablet which is cylindrical, rod and ovoid shaped and more than 8 mm in length. *e.g.* ZOLADEXTM (Goseraline Acetate Implant). DURINTM Biodegradable Implants.

Infusion Devices

1. Osmotic pressure activated drug delivery systems ALZET, DUROS infusion implant:
2. Vapour pressure activated drug delivery systems
3. Battery powered drug delivery systems

9 Pharmaceutical Aerosols

9.1 Introduction

Aerosol is a pressurized package which can be defined as a system that depends on the power of a compressed or liquefied gas to expel the contents from the container. Aerosols are unique among the pharmaceutical dosage forms because they depend on the function of a container, its valve assembly and propellants for the physical delivery of the ingredients.

Advantages

1. A dose can be removed without contamination of the remaining material.
2. Stability is enhanced for those substances adversely affected by oxygen and moisture.
3. Sterility can be maintained while a dose is being dispensed.
4. The medication can be delivered directly to the affected area in a desired form such as spray, stream, quick breaking foam or stable foam.
5. Irritation produced by the mechanical application of topical medication is reduced or eliminated.
6. Ease and convenience of application.
7. Tamper proof.
8. The physical form and the particle size of the emitted product may be controlled by proper formulation and selecting proper valve.
9. Accuracy of the administered dose.

Disadvantages

1. Precipitation of dissolved solid may occur at the administration site due to temperature differences between the content of aerosol preparation and respiratory track.

2. Some propellant causes ozone layer depletion (Choro fluoro carbon).

3. Toxicity.

4. Explosivity.

9.2 Components of Aerosol

The aerosol product essentially is a combination of gases used for dispersion of the drug packaged under high pressure in a container. The pressure inside the package is created by the presence of one or more liquefied or gaseous propellants. When the valve is actuated the pressure expel the contents through the opening in the valve.

The aerosol product consists of the following components as shown in Figure 9.1.

1. Propellants
2. Containers
3. Valves and actuators and
4. Product concentrate

9.2.1 Propellants

The propellant is generally regarded as the heart of the aerosol package which is responsible for development of pressure within the container, also expels the product when the valve is opened and aids in the atomization or foam production of the product.

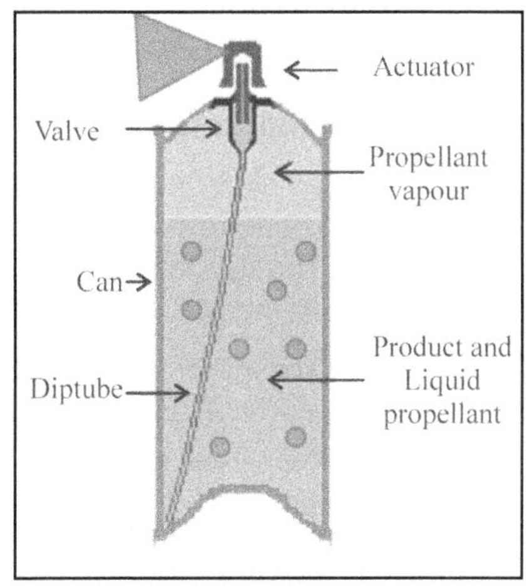

FIGURE 9.1 Components of aerosol

Various chemical compounds have been used as propellants.

9.2.1.1 Fluorinated Hydrocarbons

Fluorinated hydrocarbons also called Chloro fluoro carbons are inert, non toxic, non-inflammable and are used for oral and inhalation aerosols. Among the fluorinated hydrocarbons trichloro mono fluoro methane (Propellant 11), dichlorodi fluoro methane (Propellant 12) and dichloro tetrafluoroethane (Propellant 114) are used in oral and topical pharmaceutical aerosols. However, the depletion of ozone layer has restricted their use to oral and inhalation products.

9.2.1.2 Hydrocarbons

Topical aerosol utilized hydrocarbons such as Propane (A-108), butane (A-17), isobutane (A-31) and compressed gases such as nitrogen, carbon dioxide, and nitrous oxide. Depending on the vapor pressure and concentration of the propellant, the product is obtained in different physical forms such as sprays, mist, solid stream or foam. Usually, the combination of propellants has to be used to obtain range of vapor pressure. The vapor pressure of the mixture of propellants is calculated according to Dalton's law, which states that the total pressure in any system is equal to the sum of the individual or partial pressure of various components. Various blends of fluorinated hydro carbons are used in order to get the desired vapor pressure.

9.2.1.3 Compressed Gases

Gases such as nitrogen, nitrous oxide, and carbon dioxide have been used as aerosol propellants for products dispensed as fine mists, foams, or semisolids. But due to their low expansion ratio, the sprays are fairly wet and the foams are not as stable as produced by liquefied gas propellants.

Nomenclature of Propellant: The numerical designations for fluorinated hydrocarbon propellants have been designed so the chemical structure of the compound can be determined from the number as given in Table 9.1. The system consists of three digits.

- The digit at the extreme right refers to the number of fluorine atoms in the molecule.

- The second digit from the right represent one greater in the number of hydrogen atoms in the molecule.

- The third digit from the right is one less than the number of carbon atoms in the molecule; if this third digit is 0, it is omitted and a two-digit number is used.

- The capital letter "C" is used before a number to indicate the cyclic nature of a compound.

- The small letters following a number are used to indicate decreasing symmetry of isomeric compounds. The most symmetrical compound is given the designated number, and all other isomers are assigned a letter (i.e., a, b, etc.) in descending order of symmetry.

- The number of chlorine atoms in a molecule may be determined by subtracting the total number of hydrogen and fluorine atoms from the total number of atoms required to saturate the compound.

TABLE 9.1

Nomenclature of propellant

Name	Formula	Designated No
Tricholomono floro methane		**11**
Chloro difluoro methane	$CHClF_2$	22
Di clorotetra foro ethane		114
Trifluoromonofluoroethane	CF_3CH_2F	134a
Chlorodifluoroethane	CH_3CClF_2	142b
Difluoroethane	CH_3CHF_2	152a
Heptafluoropropane	CF_3CHFCF_3	227
Propane	C_3H_8	A-108
Isobutane	C_4H_{10}	A-31
Butane	C_4H_{10}	A17

9.2.2 Containers

Different materials are used for the manufacture of aerosol containers which must be inert, non-toxic and can withstand pressure as high as 140 to 180 pounds per square inch gauge (psig), indicating that the pressure is relative to atmospheric pressure at 130 °F.

I. Metal

   (a) **Tin-plated steel**
- Side beam (three piece)
- Two piece
- Tin free steel

   (b) **Aluminum**
- Two piece
- One piece

   (c) **Stainless steel**

II. Glass

    (a) **Unprotected**

    (b) **Plastic coated**

9.2.2.1 Metal

(a) ***Tin-plated steel:*** The tinplate steel container consists of a sheet of steel plate that has been electroplated on both the sides with tin. It is obtained in thin sheets and when required coated with an organic material. These sheets are lithographed at this point. The sheet is cut into pieces to make a body, a top and a bottom. The body is shaped into a cylinder and soldered. The top and bottom are attached to the body and a side seam stripe is added to the side seam area. The thickness of the tin coating is described in terms of its weight. A recent development in tin plate container is the welded side seam. Welding eliminates the operation of soldering, hence saves time and decreases the product container interactions. This is available in two form namely, (a) Side – seam (three pieces) and (b) Two – piece or drawn.

(b) ***Aluminium:***

(a) Two-piece

(b) One-piece (extruded or drawn)

Aluminum is used to manufacture extruded or seamless aerosol containers. Many of the pharmaceuticals are packaged in aluminum containers because of the lessened danger of in-compatibility due to its seamless nature and greater resistance to corrosion. However, aluminum can be corroded by pure water and pure ethanol. The combination of ethanol and propellant 11 in an aluminum container has been shown to produce hydrogen, acetyl chloride, aluminum chloride, propellant 21 and corrosive products. This is also available in two form namely (a) Two-piece and (b) One-piece (extruded or drawn).

(c) ***Stainless steel:*** Stainless steel containers are limited to small size because of production problems and cost. They are extremely strong and resistant to most materials. No internal organic coating is necessary.

9.2.2.2 Glass

Glass containers have been used for a large number of aerosol pharmaceuticals available with or without plastic coatings. Advantages are elimination of compatibility problems, degree of flexibility in design. The organic coatings provide added protection to the glass container. *E.g.* (A) Uncoated glass (B) Plastic – coated glass.

9.2.3 Valves

Valve must be multifunctional so that it is capable of delivering the contents in the desired form. Also in case of metered dose inhaler aerosol, the valve is expected to deliver a given amount of medication. Thus there are mainly two types of valves:

1. Continuous spray valves 2. Metering valves

9.2.3.1 Continuous Spray Valves

Typical aerosol valve assembly consists of:

(i)   Ferrule or Mounting cup

(ii) Valve body or Housing

(iii) Stem

(iv) Gasket

(v)   Spring and

(vi) Dip tube.

(i)   ***Ferrule or mounting cup***: The ferrule or mounting cup is used to attach the valve properly to the container. It is generally made from tin-plate steel or aluminum depending on the dimension of the opening of the container. To increase the resistance to corrosion a single or double epoxy or vinyl coating is added to the underside of the mounting cup.

(ii) ***Valve body or housing***: The valve body or housing is generally manufactured from nylon or Delrin. The housing has the dip tube attached at its bottom.

(iii) ***Stem***: Stem is made from nylon or Delrin, but metals such as stainless steel can be utilized. One or more orifice is set into the stem; they range from one orifice at about 0.013 inch to 0.030 inch, to three orifices of 0.040 inch each.

(iv) ***Gasket***: Gasket is made from Buna-N and Neoprene rubber and are compatible with most of the pharmaceutical formulations.

(v) *Spring*: Spring serves to hold the gasket in place and is made of stainless steel. When the actuator is depressed and released, it returns the valve to its closed position

(vi) *Dip tube*: Dip tube is made of polyethylene or polypropylene. The inside diameter varies from 0.120 inch to 0.125 inch. Viscosity and delivery rate plays an important role in the selection of the inner diameter of the dip tube.

9.2.3.2 Metering Valves

Metered valves are designed to deliver the potent medication into the nasal and respiratory airways. These operate on the principal of a chamber whose size determines the amount of drug dispensed. This reduces the number of administration errors in pharmaceutical aerosols.

9.2.4 Actuators

The actuator is a specially designed button fitted to the valve stem which delivers the

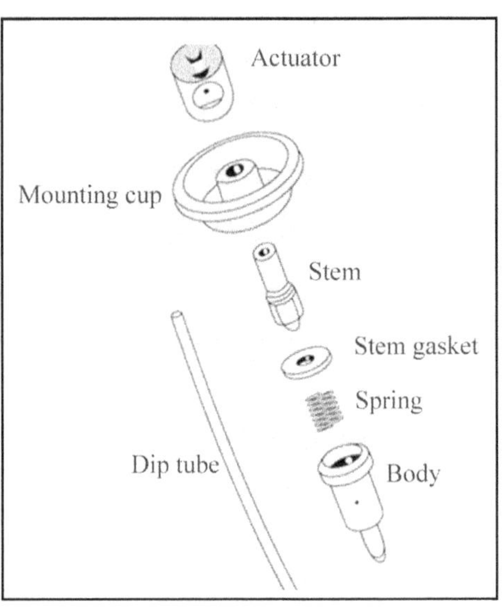

FIGURE 9.2 Valve system of aerosol.

product in a proper and a desired form. It allows easy opening and closing of the valve and is an integral part of every aerosol package. It serves to aid in producing the required type of product discharge. There are many types of actuators which may produce different forms of final product and include:

1. *Spray actuators*: are capable of dispersing the stream of product concentrate and propellant into relatively small particles by allowing the stream to pass through various openings (of which there may be one to three on the order of 0.016 inch to 0.040 inch in diameter). A spray actuator can be used for topical use such as spray on bandages, antiseptics, local anesthetic and foot preparation.

2. *Foam actuators*: consist of large orifices ranging from 0.070 to 0.128 inches. The product is dispensed into a relatively large

chamber where it can expand and is then dispersed through the large orifices. The product contains a small concentration of propellant of low vapor pressure which further aids in foam production.

3. ***Solid stream actuator***: These actuators are mainly used for ointments. They are similar to foam type. Special actuators are designed to deliver the medication to the appropriate site of action – throat, eye, and nose.

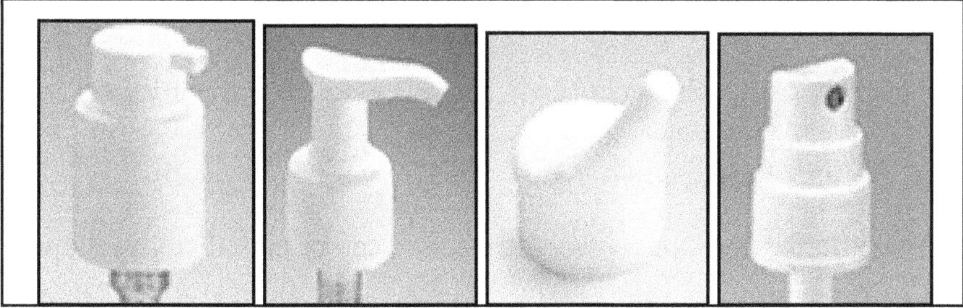

FIGURE 9.3 Various actuators for aerosols.

9.2.5 Product Concentrates

The product concentrate is the active ingredient of the aerosol in combination with the other additives such as:

- Drug
- Propellant/s: To deliver the contents from the container
- Antioxidants: to prevent from the degradation of product
- Surface active agents/ Surfactants: T o enhance miscibility or solubility
- Solvent/s: To prepare a stable and efficacious product
- Other excipients: Vehicles, suspending agents etc.

9.3   Formulation of Aerosol

An aerosol product essentially consists of two components:

1. Product concentrates
2. Propellant
1. The product concentrate consists of:

   (a) Active ingredients or mixture of active ingredients

   (b) Other necessary agents such as solvents, antioxidants and surfactants.

2. The propellant may be single propellant or a blend of various propellants to give the desired vapor pressure.

The pharmaceutical aerosol may be dispensed as a fine mist, wet spray, and quick – breaking foam, stable foam, (semi-solid or solid). The type of system selected depends on many factors:

1. Physical, chemical and pharmacological properties of active ingredients and

2. Site of application

The different types of aerosol formulation can be classified as follows:

1. Solution system or Two phase system

2. Water-based system or Three phase system

3. Suspension or dispersion systems

4. Foam systems

   (a) Stable foam

   (b) Aqueous stable foam

   (c) Non aqueous stable foam

   (d) Quick breaking foam

   (e) Intranasal aerosols.

9.3.1 Solution System

A large number of aerosols can be formulated as a solution system which consists of two phases: a vapor phase and a liquid phase. Here the active ingredient is soluble in the propellant and thus forms a solution of the drug or active ingredient. Depending on the type of spray required, the propellant consist of:

   (i) Propellant 12 or A-70 (which provides very fine particles because of higher vapor pressure).

   (ii) A mixture of propellant 12 and other propellants. If the other propellants have lower vapor pressure, the pressure of the final system decreases resulting in larger particles. Also lowering of the vapor pressure is produced through the addition of less volatile solvents such as ethyl alcohol, propylene glycol, ethyl acetate, glycerin and acetone. These are solvents added to increase the solubility of drug in the propellant. The amount of propellant used may vary from 5% for foams to 95% for inhalation products of the entire formulation. Spray systems with large particles are also useful topical preparations, since they tend to coat the affected area with a film of active ingredients.

9.3.2 Water Based Systems

Also known as three phase system, contain large amounts of water added to replace all or part of the non aqueous solvent used in aerosol. Depending on the formulation, they are emitted as a spray or foam to produce a spray, the formulation must consist of dispersed drugs and other solvents in an emulsion system in which the propellant is in the external phase. In this way, when the product is dispensed, the propellant vaporizes and dispenses the active ingredients into minute particles. Since propellant water are mostly not miscible, a three phase aerosol forms (propellant phase, water and vapor phase). The difference between the Aquasol system and the 'three phase system' is that the former dispenses a dry spray with very small particles and the latter dispensed a wet spray.

9.3.3 Suspension or Dispersion Systems

Various methods have been used to overcome the disadvantages of using co-solvent specially alcohol which is flammable and causes chilling sensation. One method is to suspend or disperse the drug in a propellant or mixture of propellants to prevent or decrease the rate of settling of disperse particles, various surfactants or suspending agents are added to the system. These systems have been developed for use with oral inhalation aerosol.

9.3.4 Foam Systems

Foam systems are mainly used for external preparations and not used for pulmonary delivery. Emulsion and foam aerosols consist of active ingredients, aqueous or non-aqueous vehicle, surfactant and propellant and are dispersed as stable or quick breaking foam depending on the nature of the ingredients and the formulation.

(a) *Aqueous stable foams***:** Aqueous stable foams contain water as the vehicle. In order to impart stability to the formulation, a large concentration of lipids are incorporated as oil in water emulsion.

(b) *Non aqueous stable foams***:** Non-aqueous stable foams are formulated by the use of polyethylene glycol.

(c) *Quick-breaking foams***:** The propellant is present in low concentration and in the external phase. When the product is dispensed it is emitted as foam which immediately collapses into liquid.

(d) *Thermal foams***:** These systems were developed early to produce warm foam for shaving. These systems would be advantageous in dispensing medicaments in which application of heat is desirable.

9.3.5 Intranasal Aerosols

Drug delivery systems intended for the deposition of medication into the nasal passageways have been used for long time as an effective means of administering drugs intended to produce either local or systemic effect. These would offer various advantages such as, delivery of measured dose of drug, excellent depth penetration into the nasal passage ways, reduced droplets size, lower dose, and maintenance of sterility.

The major difference between inhalation and intranasal product is the design of the adaptor. The nasal adaptor is shorter, narrower and minimization of propellant vaporization before contacting the mucosa.

9.4   Manufacture of Aerosol

The manufacture of aerosol products takes place in two stages:

1. Manufacture of the concentrate and

2. Filling of the propellant

The aerosol concentrate consists of drug or combination of drugs, solvents, antioxidants and surfactants formulated as solution, suspension or foam systems. The aerosol concentrate is first prepared and filled into the container. The propellant is then filled into the container. Therefore, part of the manufacturing operation takes place during the filling operation which requires special quality control measures to ensure that both concentrate and propellant are brought together in the proper proportion. Filling operation is a unique step specific for aerosol products.

The equipments used for manufacture of aerosols can be classified into two classes:

1. Equipments used for compounding of liquids, suspensions, emulsions, creams and ointments.
2. Specialized equipments capable of handling and packaging materials at relatively low temperatures (above –40 °F) or under high pressure.

Three methods have been developed for filling of aerosol products:

9.4.1 Cold Filling Method

The principle of cold filling method requires the chilling of all components including concentrate and propellant to a temperature of –30° to –40° F. The propellant liquefies when chilled. First, the product concentrate is chilled and filled into already chilled container followed by the chilled liquefied propellant.

Advantages

1. Easy process.
2. System can be used with metered as well as non metered valve.

Disadvantages

1. Chilling of the product, container and propellant is required.
2. Aqueous products, emulsions and those products adversely affected by cold temperature cannot be filled by this method.
3. Loss of propellant during air evacuation.

9.4.2 Pressure Filling Process

Pressure filling is carried out at room temperature under high pressure. The apparatus consists of a pressure burette capable of metering small volumes of liquefied gas under pressure into an aerosol container. The propellant is added through the inlet valve located at the bottom or top of the burette. Trapped air is allowed to escape through the upper valve. The desired amount of propellant is allowed to flow through the aerosol valve into the container under its own vapor pressure. When the pressure is equalized between the burette and the container (thus happens with low pressure propellant), the propellant stops flowing. To help in adding additional propellant, a hose leading to a cylinder of nitrogen or compressed gas is attached to the upper valve and the added nitrogen pressure causes the propellant to flow.

Advantages

1. No refrigeration is required. It is the preferred method because some solutions, emulsions, suspensions and other preparations cannot be chilled.
2. Lesser danger of contamination of product with the moisture.
3. Less propellant is lost.

9.4.3 Compressed Gas Filling

Compressed gases are present under high pressure in cylinders. These cylinders are fitted with a pressure reducing valve and a delivery gauge. The delivery gauge is in turn fitted with flexible hose capable of withstanding about 150 lbs per square inch gauge pressure and a filling head.

Advantages

1. Easy process.
2. Can be carried out at Room temperature.

Disadvantages

Compressed gas is used as a propellant in topical preparations and not used in oral inhalation products used for pulmonary delivery.

9.5   Stability Testing of Aerosols

A stability program for aerosol formulation consists of an examination of all materials used in the product both separately and collectively. The parameters to be evaluated depending on the type of product to be evaluated and include:

1. ***Metered dose inhalers, oral and nasal aerosols***: Pressure, weight loss, total medication, can content, weight uniformity, moisture content, valve delivery, particle size, unit spray, degraded product, content uniformity, particulate matter and interaction of product with can should be evaluated.
2. ***Topical sprays pressure***: Weight loss, delivery rate, specific gravity, density, viscosity, interaction of the product with valve, interaction

of product with containers, and other depending upon on the nature of the product need to be evaluated in this type of aerosol.

3. *Foams*: Same as sprays, foam density and characteristics, amount delivered if metered, amount delivered if non-metered are the characters which are needed to be evaluated.

   The effect of container on the product and the effect of product on the container and the value and dip tube must be studied. All materials must be studied separately and collectively.

4. *Valve/Dip tube*: Should be examined to ensure that it is functional and easily dispense the product and can be easily closed. The valve cup should be examined for corrosion, softening, cracking, elongation or distortion. Elongation and cracking of the dip tube should be checked.

9.6   Quality Control Tests for Aerosols

The quality control of aerosol includes, the testing of Raw materials (propellants, valves, actuators, dip tube, and containers) and Testing during Manufacturing (Weight, leak and spray testing).

9.6.1 Specifications for Raw Materials

9.6.1.1 Propellants

1. Determining its vapour pressure and should be compared to specifications.
2. Determining its density and should be compared to specifications.
3. Identity is determined by gas chromatography as well as to determine the composition of the blend of propellants.
4. Purity and acceptability of propellants is tested by moisture, halogen and non-volatile residue determinations.

9.6.1.2 Valves, Actuators and Dip Tubes

These parts are subjected to both physical and chemical inspection. Additional tests on the valve to ensure that the valves are fit to be used. These tests include using specific test solution and procedure for acceptance of the valve.

9.6.1.3 Containers

Both uncoated and coated metal containers are examined for defects in the lining. Glass containers are examined for flaws. The dimensions of the neck and other parts are checked to determine conformity to specifications. The weight of the container is also checked.

9.6.2 Testing during Manufacture

(a) *Weight checking*: Weight checking is carried out periodically, by adding a tared empty aerosol contains to the filling line. After it is filled with concentrate and accurately weighed. The same procedure is adopted to check the weight of the propellant that is being added. As a further check, the finished container is weighed to check the accuracy of the filling operation.

(b) *Leak testing*: It done by checking the crimping of the valve to ensure that there are no defective containers. The efficiency of the valve closure is made by passing the filled containers through a heated water bath kept at 130 °F.

(c) *Spray testing*: All aerosols are 100% spray tested and checked for defects in the valve and the spray pattern.

9.6.3 Testing of Finished Product

Tests have been designed to ensure proper performance of the package and safety during use and storage. Thus pharmaceutical aerosols can be evaluated by a series of physical, chemical and biological tests including.

9.6.3.1 Flammability and Combustibility

(a) *Flame projection*: This test indicates the effect of an aerosol formulation on the extension of an open flame. The product is sprayed for about 4 seconds into a flame. Depending on the nature of formulations, the flame is extended, the exact length being measured with a ruler.

(b) *Flash Point*: This is determined by use of a standard 'Tag Open Cup Apparatus'. The aerosol product is chilled to a temperature of -25 °F and transferred to the test apparatus. The test liquid is allowed to increase slowly in temperature, and the temperature at which the vapors ignite is taken as the flash point.

9.6.3.2 Physicochemical Characteristics

(a) *Vapor pressure*: Measured by using a pressure gauge. If pressure variation from container to container is excessive, it indicates the pressure of air is present in the headspace.

(b) ***Density***: Accurately determined by using a hydrometer or pycnometer.

(c) ***Moisture content***: Determined by using Karl Fisher or Gas Chromatographic methods.

(d) ***Identification of propellants***: Gas chromatography and Infrared Spectrophotometry are used to identify the propellant and also to indicate the proportion of each component in blend.

(e) ***Particle size determination***: Many methods have been developed to determine the particle size among the methods; the most extensively used are the cascade impactor and 'light scatter decay' methods. Cascade impactor operates on the principle that in a stream of particles projected through a series of nozzles and glass slides at high velocity, the larger particles become impacted first on the lower velocity stages and the smaller particles pass on and are collected at higher velocity stages.

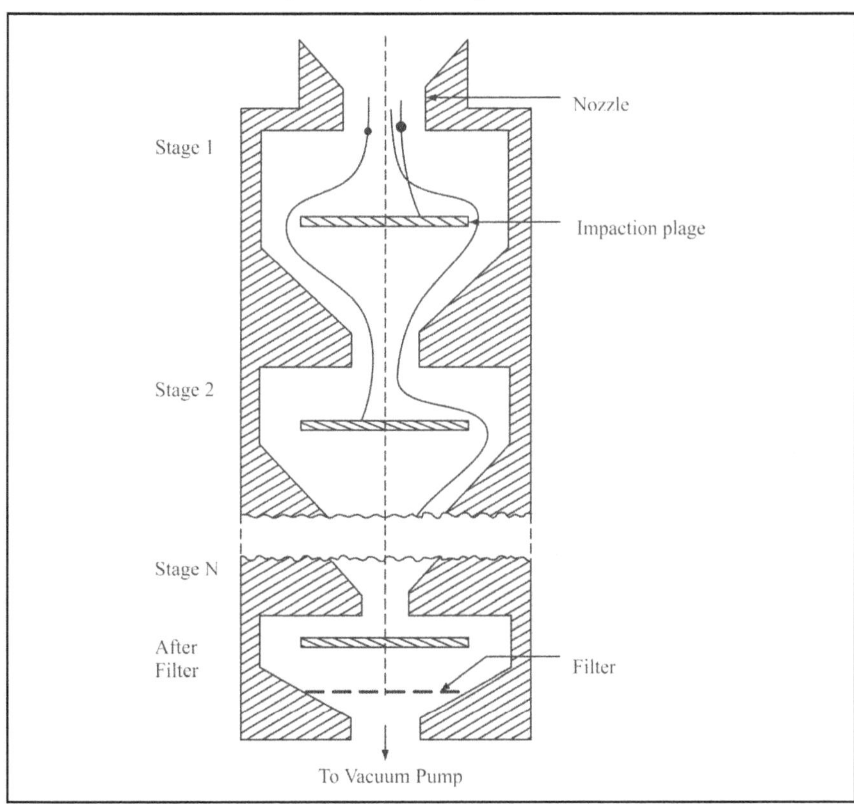

FIGURE 9.4 The cascade impactor.

9.6.3.3 Performance

(a) *Aerosol valve discharge rate*: This is determined by taking an aerosol product and weighing it initially. The contents are discharged for a given period of time using standard apparatus. The container is reweighed after a particular period of time. Change in weight per unit time gives the aerosol valve discharge rate usually expressed as grams per second.

(b) *Spray pattern*: Spray Pattern is determined and compared with the spray pattern obtained from different batches of material to ensure uniformity from batch to batch. Also spray pattern may be characteristic of the valve used. The method used to determine the pattern is based on the impingement of the spray on a piece of a paper that has been treated with a dye-talc mixture. Depending on the nature of aerosol, an oil-soluble or water-soluble dye is used. The particles that strike the paper cause the dye to go into the solution and to be absorbed onto the paper. This gives a record of the spray, which can be used for comparison purposes. To control the amount of material coming into contact with the paper, the paper is attached to a rotating disk that has an adjustable slit which controls the amount of material that falls on the paper.

(c) *Reproducibility of dosage*: Reproducibility of dosage determined by dispensing one or more dose into a solvent in which the drug is soluble. The solution of drug is then assayed and amount of active ingredients determined. Another method that can be used to measure reproducibility involves accurate weighing of filled container, followed by dispensing of several doses. The container is then reweighed, and the difference in weight divided by the number of doses dispensed gives the average dose. This test must be repeated and results compared.

(d) *Net contents*: Several methods have been developed to determine if sufficient product has been placed into each container

   1. The tarred cans are placed into the filling line, after being accurately weighed, difference in weight is equal to the net contents.

   2. Another is a destructive method and consists of weighing a full container and then dispensing the contents. The container is reweighed after making provision for the amount of remaining material in the container, the net content in each container is determined.

(e) *Foam stability*: Several methods have been used, which include a visual evaluation, time for a given mass to penetrate the foam, time for a given rod that is inserted into the foam to fall and use of rotational viscometers.

9.6.3.4 Biological Testing

Many biological tests have been used to evaluate the efficiency of many products, including various antibacterial agents. These tests are explained in therapeutic efficacy and toxicity studies.

(a) *Therapeutic efficacy or activity*: Various testing procedures are available to determine the therapeutic activity of aerosols. The procedures are similar to the non-aerosols. e.g. topical preparations are applied to the test areas and adsorption of therapeutic ingredient is determined.

(b) *Toxicity*: Toxicity testing should include both in topical and inhalation effects. Aerosols applied topically may be irritating to the affected area and or may cause a chilling effect. The degree of chilling depends on the type and amount of propellant present. Inhalation toxicity must be considered even though the product may be intended for topical administration. This can be accomplished by exposing test animals to vapours sprayed from an aerosol container.

9.7 Advancements in Aerosol System

- *Pressurized metered dose inhalers*: A metered dose inhaler is device that delivers a specific amount of medication in aerosol form. There is a breakthrough development in various types of valve holding chambers or spacers. Spacers are particularly important for steroid inhalation to maximize lung deposition and minimize unwanted oropharyngeal deposition.

- *Dry powder inhalers*: It is a device that delivers medication to the lungs in the form of a dry powder.

- *Breath actuated inhalers*: Breath-actuated inhalers are inhalers that automatically release a spray of medication when the person begins to inhale.

10 Ophthalmic Preparations

10.1 Introduction

Ophthalmic preparations are sterile products that are intended to be applied to the eyelids or placed in the space between the eyelids and the eyeball.

The eye is a unique organ from anatomical and physiological point of view. It contains several different structures with specific physiological functions. The human eye has a spherical shape with a diameter of 23 mm. The structural components of the eyeball are divided into three layers: the outermost coat comprises of a clear, transparent cornea and the white, opaque sclera; the middle layer comprises the iris anteriorly, the choroids posteriorly, the ciliary body; and the inner layer is the retina, which is an extension of the central nervous system. The cornea and the crystalline lens are the only tissues in the body in addition to cartilage which have no blood supply, whereas choroid and ciliary processes are highly vascularized and exhibit very high blood flows. The retina with the optic nerve, an extension of the diencephalon of the central nervous system, has a very specific function in the visual perception and transduction phenomena. Ocular disposition and elimination of a therapeutic agent is dependent upon its physicochemical properties as well as the relevant ocular anatomy and physiology.

The cornea is often the tissue through which drugs in ophthalmic preparations reach the inside of the eye. Because the structure of the cornea consists of epithelium stroma, which is equivalent to a fat–water–fat structure, the penetration of nonpolar compounds through the cornea depends on their oil/water partition coefficients. The fluid systems in the eye - the aqueous humor and the vitreous humor also play an important role in ocular pharmacokinetics. The aqueous humor fills the anterior and posterior chambers of the eye and is secreted continuously from the blood through the epithelium of the ciliary body. When a drug is instilled into the eye, there exists a large number of factors that can influence its distribution and movement into various parts of the eye or the body as a whole. Topically applied ocular drugs may be intended to exert a local effect or to penetrate into the anterior chamber to be distributed to various eye tissues.

Advantages of ocular drug delivery systems

1. Increased accurate dosing. To overcome the side effects of pulsed dosing produced by conventional systems.
2. To provide sustained and controlled drug delivery.
3. To increase the ocular bioavailability of drug by increasing the corneal contact time. This can be achieved by effective adherence to corneal surface.
4. To provide targeting within the ocular globe so as to prevent the loss to other ocular tissues.
5. To circumvent the protective barriers like drainage, lacrimation and conjunctival absorption.
6. To provide comfort, better compliance to the patient and to improve therapeutic performance of drug.
7. To provide better housing of delivery system.

Limitations of ophthalmic drug delivery

1. Dosage form cannot be terminated during emergency.
2. Interference with vision.
3. Difficulty in placement and removal.
4. Occasional loss during sleep or while rubbing eyes.

10.2 Anatomy and Physiology of Eye

The eye is a spherical structure with a wall consisting of three layers; the outer sclera, the middle choroid layer, ciliary body, iris and the inner nervous tissue layer retina as shown in Figure 10.1.

- ***Sclera***: The protective outer layer of the eye, referred to as the "white of the eye" and it maintains the shape of the eye.

- ***Choroid*:** The choroid is the second layer of the eye and lies between the sclera and the retina. It contains the blood vessels that provide nourishment to the outer layers of the retina.

- ***Cornea*:** The front portion of the sclera, is transparent and allows light to enter the eye. The cornea is a powerful refracting surface, providing much of the eye's focusing power. It is a vascular tissue to which nutrient and oxygen are supplied via bathing with lachrymal fluid and aqueous humour as well as from blood vessels that lines the junction between the cornea and sclera.

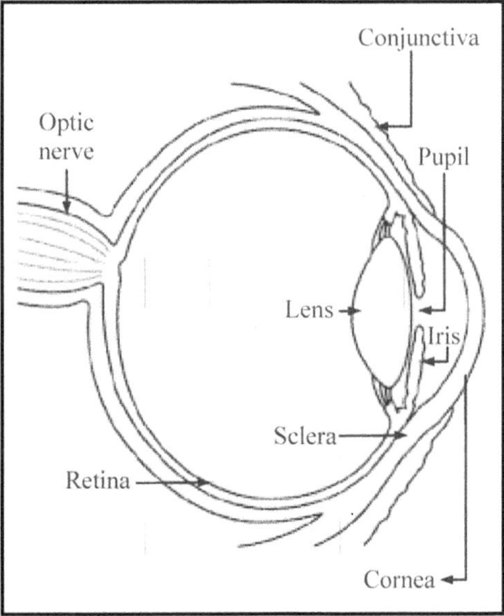

FIGURE 10.1 Anatomy of eye.

- ***It is composed of five layers*:** Epithelium, Bowman's layer, stroma, Descemet's membrane and endothelium. The epithelium consists of 5 to 6 layers of cells. The epithelium is squamous stratified, consisting of 5-6 layer of cells with a total thickness around 50-100 μm and turnover of about one cell layer per day.

- ***Iris*:** The iris is the part of the eye that gives it color. The iris is a diaphragm of variable size whose function is to adjust the size of the pupil to regulate the amount of light admitted into the eye.

- ***Retina*:** The retina is the innermost layer in the eye. It converts images into electrical impulses that are sent along the optic nerve to the brain where the images are interpreted.

- ***Lens*:** The lens is a transparent, biconvex structure, encased in a thin transparent covering. The function of the lens is to refract and focus incoming light onto the retina.

- ***The macula*:** is located in the back of the eye, in the center of the retina. This area produces the sharpest vision.

- ***Conjunctiva*:** The conjunctiva is a mucous membrane that begins at the edge of the cornea and lines the inside surface of the eyelids and sclera, which serves to lubricate the eye. The conjunctiva is involved in the formation and maintenance of the precorneal tear film and in the protection of the eye.

- *Pupil*: Pupil generally appears to be the dark "centre" of the eye, but can be more accurately described as the circular aperture in the centre of the iris through which light passes into the eye.

- *Ciliary Muscle*: The ciliary muscle is a ring of striated smooth muscles in the eye's middle layer that controls accommodation for viewing objects at varying distances and regulates the flow of aqueous humour into schlemm's canal.

- *Aqueous humour*: The aqueous humour is a jelly-like substance located in the outer/front chamber of the eye. It is a watery fluid that fills the "anterior chamber of the eye" which is located immediately behind the cornea and in front of the lens.

- *Vitreous humour*: The vitreous humour (also known as the vitreous body) is located in the large area that occupies approximately 80% of each eye in the human body. The vitreous humour is a perfectly transparent thin-jelly-like substance that fills the chamber behind the lens of the eye.

10.3 Mechanism of Ocular Drug Absorption

Drugs administered by instillation in the type must penetrate the eye and do so primarily through the cornea followed by the non-corneal routes. These non-corneal routes involve drug diffusion across the conjunctiva and sclera and appear to be particularly important for drugs that are poorly absorbed across the cornea as shown in Figure 10.2.

10.3.1 Occular Bioavailability

Physiological factors that can affect a drugs ocular bioavailability are protein binding, drug metabolism, lachrymal drainage, physiochemical characteristics of drug and types of product formulation. The various constraints for occular absorption of drugs includes solution drainage, tear dilution, tear turnover, blinking reflexes and conjunctival absorption. Drug solution drainage from the precorneal area is the most significant factor in reducing the ocular contact time and is bioavailability of solution dosage forms. The instilled dose leaves within 5 minutes and is rapidly lost through naso-lacrimal drainage. The drug, the pH, and the tonicity of the dosage forms can induce lacrimation. Normal human tear turnover is 16% per minute and it also contributes to remove drug solution from the conjunctival cul-de-sac.

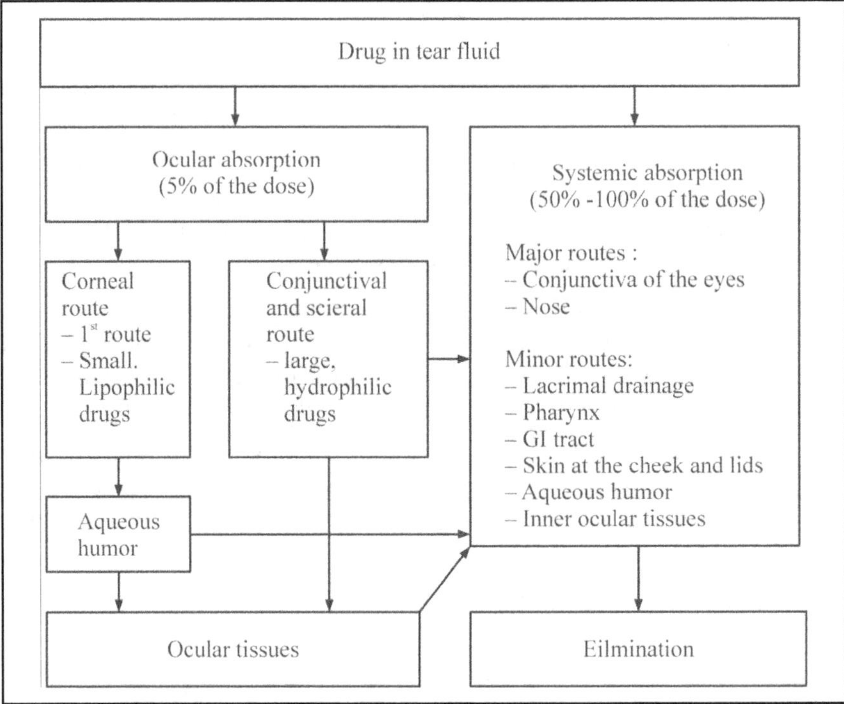

FIGURE 10.2 Mechanism of ocular drug absorption.

10.4 Classification of Ocular Drug Delivery Systems

A multitude of ocular dosage forms are available for delivery of drugs to the eye. These can be classified on the basis of their physical forms as follows:

1. ***Liquids*:** Solutions, Suspensions, Sol to gel systems, Sprays.

2. ***Solids*:** Ocular inserts, Contact lenses, Corneal shield, Artificial tear inserts, Filter paper strips.

3. ***Semi-solids*:** Ointments, Gels.

4. ***Miscellaneous*:** Ocular iontophoresis, Vesicular systems, Mucoadhesive dosage forms, Particulates, Ocular penetration enhancers.

10.4.1 Solutions

Ophthalmic solutions are sterile solutions intended for instillation into the eye. Solution should remain in the eye in order to produce the desired therapeutic effect. Ophthalmic solutions usually do not impair or interfere with the vision of the patient. Preparation of an ophthalmic solution requires careful consideration of factors like the inherent toxicity of the drug, isotonicity, buffering, preservation, sterilization and proper packaging.

10.4.2 Suspensions

Ophthalmic suspensions are sterile liquid preparations containing solid particles dispersed in a liquid vehicle intended for application to the eye. Suspensions should contain the drug in a micronized form to prevent irritation and scratching of the cornea. suspensions produce a longer effect than solutions do.

10.4.3 Ophthalmic Ointments

Ophthalmic ointments are semisolid preparations which are easy to apply and remain in contact with the eye tissues for an extended period. Hence, they usually produce a therapeutic effect for longer duration. One major disadvantage of ointments is that they leave a film over the patient's eye which leads to vision impairment.

10.4.4 Ocular Inserts

Ocular inserts are defined as sterile solid or semisolid preparations, with a thin, flexible and multilayered structure, for insertion in the conjunctival sac. The ocular inserts maintain an effective drug concentration in the target tissues and minimizes the number of applications.

Advantages

- Increasing contact time and improving bioavailability.
- Providing a prolong drug release and thus a better efficacy.
- Reduction of adverse effects.
- Reduction of the number administrations and thus better patient compliance.

Disadvantages

Ocular inserts have been attributed to psychological factors, such as reluctance of patients to abandon the traditional medications, and to occasional therapeutic failures.

Ocular inserts are available as erodible, nonerodible, and hydrogel inserts

- ***Erodable inserts*:** It consists of all monolytic polymeric devices that at the end of their release, the device dissolve or erode.

  Advantages

  Being entirely soluble so that they do not need to be removed from their site of application

  E.g: Lacrisert, SODI and Minidisc.

- ***Nonerodable inserts*:** It is a multilayered structure consisting of a drug containing core surrounded on each side by a layer of copolymer membranes through which the drug diffuses at a constant rate.

  E.g: Ocusert, Pilo-20 and Pilo-40 Ocular system.

10.4.5   Contact Lenses

Contact lenses can absorb water soluble drugs when soaked in drug solutions. These drug saturated contact lenses are placed in the eye for releasing the drug for long period of time. The hydrophilic contact lenses can be used to prolong the ocular residence time of the drugs. In humans, the bionite lens which are made from hydrophilic polymer (2-hydroxy ethyl methacrylate) have been shown to produce a greater penetration of fluorescein.

- ***Hard Contact Lenses:*** These are made of rigid plastic resin polymethyl methacrylate and are impermeable to oxygen and moisture.

- ***Soft Contact Lenses*:** Soft contact lenses are made of soft, flexible plastics (hydroxyl ethyl methacrylate) that Contain 30-80% water so are permeable to oxygen.

- ***Rigid Gas Permeable (RGP) Contact Lenses*:** Rigid gas permeable (RGPs) contact lenses are more durable and resistant to deposit buildup. Taking the advantages of both soft and hard lenses, they are hydrophobic and oxygen permeable.

10.5 Formulation Considerations

10.5.1 Required Characteristics of Ophthalmic Preparations

1. Ophthalmic solutions must be sterile

2. Ophthalmic solutions should be isotonic

3. Ophthalmic solutions must be sparkling clear and free of particulate matter for comfort and safety.

10.5.2 Manufacturing Process

The manufacturing processes should meet the requirements of Good Manufacturing Practices, especially with regard to cross-contamination. In process control, during production of ophthalmic preparations should include monitoring environmental conditions (especially with respect to particulate and microbial contamination), pyrogens pH and clarity of solution, and integrity of container (absence of leakage, etc.). Appropriate limits should be set for the particle size of the active ingredient. It is essential that ophthalmic preparations are sterile.

10.5.3 Ointment Bases

Ophthalmic semisolids frequently contain vehicles like soft petrolatum, absorption base and a water soluble base. Base used for topical ocular delivery falls into two general categories:

Simple bases: Simple bases refer to a single continuous phase. These include white petrolatum, lanolin and viscous gels prepared from polymers such as PVA, carbopol etc.

Compound bases: These are usually of a biphasic type forming either water in oil or oil in water emulsions.

A drug in either a simple or compound base provide an increase in the duration of action due to reduction in dilution by tears, reduction in drainage and prolonged corneal contact time. The ointment base that is selected must be impalpable to avoid eye discomfort and irritation. It should permit easy diffusion of the drug and retain the activity of the medicament for a reasonable period under proper storage conditions.

10.6   Pharmaceutical Requirements

10.6.1   Isotonicity Value

Lacrimal fluid is isotonic with blood, having an isotonicity value corresponding to that of a 0.9% sodium chloride solution. The isotonicity limits of an ophthalmic solution in terms of sodium chloride may range from solution 0.6 to 2.0% without marked discomfort. All the active and inactive components of an ophthalmic preparation, contribute to the osmotic pressure of a solution. Some ophthalmic solutions are necessarily hypertonic in order to enhance absorption. Where the amount of such solutions used is small, dilution with lacrimal fluid takes place rapidly so that discomfort from the hypertonicity is only temporary. However, any adjustment toward isotonicity by dilution with tears is negligible.

10.6.2   Buffering

The purpose of buffering ophthalmic preparation may be to render the formulation to be more stable, to enhance the aqueous solubility of the drug, to enhance the bioavailability of drug, to maximize preservative efficacy and for greater comfort to the eyes. Normal tears have a pH of about 7.4 and possess some buffer capacity. The application of a medicated solution stimulates the flow of tears which neutralizes any excess hydrogen or hydroxyl ions introduced with the solution. Ideally, an ophthalmic solution should have the same pH, as well as the same isotonicity value, as lacrimal fluid. This is not usually possible since, at pH 7.4, many drugs are not appreciably soluble in water. Most alkaloidal salts precipitate as the free alkaloid at this pH. Additionally many drugs are chemically unstable at pH levels approaching 7.4. This instability is more marked at the high temperatures employed in heat sterilization. For this reason, the buffer system should be selected that is nearest to the physiological pH of 7.4 and does not cause precipitation of the drug or its rapid deterioration.

The pH of the solution greatly effects the absorption by the eye. It is found that absorption of a 1% atropine solution at pH 4.0 is only a third as great as it is at pH 7.5. A change in pH from 4.0 to 7.5 decreased the absorption of 0.5% pilocarpine by 50%. It has also been shown that changing the pH of 1% cocaine solution from 3.2 to 8.7 increased its absorption sevenfold.

Many drugs, when buffered to a therapeutically acceptable pH, would not be stable in solution for long periods of time. for this reason, a compromise pH is selected for a solution and maintained by buffers to permit the therapeutic activity while maintaining stability. Examples of buffering vehicles are Boric acid vehicle (pH 4.7) and phosphate acid vehicles (pH 5.9-8)

10.6.3 Sterility and Preservation

Ophthalmic preparations must be sterilized for safe use. To maintain sterility during use, antimicrobial preservatives are included in ophthalmic preparation which must demonstrate safety, stability and compatibility with other formulation additives and packaging components. The most commonly used antimicrobial agents and their concentrations are given in Table 10.1

TABLE 10.1

Antimicrobial agents

Antimicrobial agents	Effective concentration (%)
Benzalkonium chloride	0.004-0.01
Benzathonium chloride	0.01
Chlorobutanol	0.5
Phenylmercuric nitrate/acetate	0.004
Thiomerosol	0.005-0.01

10.6.4 Viscosity and Thickening Agent

A pharmaceutical grade of methylcellulose (for viscosity 25 cp-1%, or 4000 cp - 0.25%) or other suitable thickening agents such as hydroxypropyl methylcellulose or polyvinyl alcohol are added to ophthalmic solutions to increase the viscosity and prolong contact of the drug with the tissue. The thickened ophthalmic solution must be free from visible particles. Viscosity for ophthalmic solutions is considered optimal in the range of 15-25 cp.

10.6.5 Stability

The stability of ophthalmic preparations during prolonged storage, and the effects of heat sterilization processes must be considered during formulation. The effects of temperature and pH are particularly important. Buffering certain drugs in the physiological pH range makes them unstable, particularly at high temperatures. Most of the common ophthalmic drugs however, in 2% boric acid solution can be autoclaved without seriously affecting their therapeutic activity. The oxidative discoloration of many drugs such as physostigmine, epinephrine and phenylephrine may be reduced by the addition of 0.2% sodium bisulphate to the vehicle. The stability of solutions is especially important, since it is found that a 44% decomposition of 0.5% atropine solution and 89% decomposition of a 1% homatropine solution in one month when they were dispensed at pH 8.3. Deterioration was found to be reduced to 20% at pH 6.8. In general, slightly acid solutions of ophthalmic drugs are more stable and effective. If they are too acidic, the free base is quite irritating. Other medications may be used at a higher pH because their bases are less irritating.

10.7   Evaluation

Ophthalmic preparations must meet the requirements of sterility. If the specific ingredients used in the formulation do not lend themselves to routine sterilization techniques, ingredients that meet the sterility requirements should be used. The finished ointment must be free from large particles and must meet the requirements for leakage and for metal particles. The immediate containers for ophthalmic ointments shall be sterile at the time of filling and closing. It is requisite that the immediate containers for ophthalmic preparations must be sealed and tamper-proof to ensure sterility at the time of use.

10.7.1   Appearance/Clarity Test

Inspect the ointments, aqueous or oily solutions, suspensions or emulsions. All the formulations should be checked for general appearance i.e., colour, odour, any suspended particulate matter etc. Evidence of physical and/or chemical instability is demonstrated by noticeable changes in colour and odour. The clarity is checked using wooden board with black and white background. The vials are held horizontally and gently rotated immediately under the lamp and then inverted once or twice to detect foreign particles.

10.7.2   Rheological Studies

Viscosity of the instilled formulation is an important factor in determining residence time of drug in the eye. The prepared solutions were allowed to gel in the simulated tear fluid and then the viscosity determination tests were carried out by using Brookfield viscometer.

10.7.3 Determination of pH

The pH of each formulation is recorded using a digital pH meter.

10.7.4 Sterility Test

Tests for sterility are adequately designed to reveal the presence of microorganisms in the samples used in the tests. Ophthalmic preparations should comply with the test for sterility. The sterility of each sterilized batch of medium is determined by incubating a portion of the media at the specified incubation temperature for 14 days. No growth of microorganisms should occur. Two well-recognized and universally accepted methods adopted are

(a) Membrane Filtration

(b) Direct Inoculation of the cultural media.

Membrane Filtration: The solution of the product under investigation is carefully filtered via a hydrophobic-edged membrane filter that would precisely retain any possible contaminating microorganisms. The resulting membrane is duly washed *in situ* to get rid of any possible 'traces of antibiotic' that would have been sticking to the surface of the membrane intimately. Finally, the segregated microorganisms are meticulously transferred to the suitable culture media under perfect aseptic environment. The membrane filtration must be used for such products where the volume in a container is either 100 ml or more.

Direct Inoculation of the Cultural Media: The three usual methods being used for performing the 'tests for sterility' are

(a) Nutrient Broth,
(b) Cooked meat medium and thioglycollate medium, and
(c) Sabouraud medium.

10.7.5 Leak Test

Ten tubes of the ointment with seal placed in a horizontal position on a sheet of absorbent blotting paper in an oven maintained at a temperature of 60 ± 3 °C for 8 hours. For any tube no significant leakage should occur during or at the completion of the test. If leakage is observed from one, but not more than one, of the tubes, the test is repeated with 20 additional tubes of the ointment. The requirement is met if no leakage is observed from the first 10 tubes tested, or if leakage is observed from not more than one of 30 tubes tested.

10.7.6   Uniform Consistency

Ophthalmic ointments should be of uniform consistency. When a sample is rubbed on the back of the hand, no solid components should be noticed.

10.7.7   Metal Particle in Ophthalmic Preparation

This test is designed to limit a level of unobjectionable number and size of discrete metal particles that may occur in ophthalmic ointments.

Extrude, the contents of 10 tubes individually into separate, clear, flat-bottom, petri dishes that are free from scratches. Cover the dishes and heat at 85 °C for 2 hours. Then allow each to cool to room temperature and to solidify.

Remove the covers, and invert each Petri dish on the stage of a suitable microscope equipped with an eye-piece micrometer. Examine the entire bottom of the petri dish for metal particles. Varying the intensity of the illuminator from above allows such metal particles to be recognized by their characteristic reflection of light. Count the number of metal particles that are 50μm or larger in any dimension. The requirements are met if the total number of such particles in all 10 tubes does not exceed 50, and if not more than one tube is found to contain more than 8 such particles. If these results fail, repeat the test on 20 additional tubes, the requirements are met if the total number of metal particles that are 50 μm or larger in any dimension does not exceed 150 in all 30 tubes tested, and if not more than 3 of the tubes are found to contain more than 8 such particles each.

10.7.8   Accelerated Stability Studies

Formulation is stored at 40 °C and 75% RH and 25 °C and 60% RH for a period of 3 months. The formulation was evaluated at periodic intervals for drug content, clarity, pH, sol–gel transition, rheology, *in vitro* drug release and sterility.

10.8 Storage and Packaging of Ophthalmic Preparations

Ophthalmic preparations should maintain their integrity throughout their shelf-life when stored at the temperature indicated on the label. If not otherwise stated, the storage temperature should not exceed 25 °C. Special storage recommendations or limitations are indicated in individual monographs. Packaging must be adequate to protect ophthalmic preparations from light, moisture, microbial contamination, and damage due to handling and transportation.

The final container should be appropriate for the ophthalmic product and its intended use and should not interfere with the stability and efficacy of the preparation. Ophthalmic liquids can be packaged in sterile plastic bottles with self-contained dropper tips or in glass bottles with separate droppers. Ophthalmic solutions and suspensions are commonly packaged in 2, 2.5, 5, 10, 15 and 30 mL of product. Ophthalmic ointments are generally packed in a metal container with an epoxy or vinyl plastic coating. A large volume intraocular preparation (Irrigation) may be packaged in a glass or polyolefin containers. Containers, including the closures, for ophthalmic ointments should not interact physically or chemically with the preparation to alter the strength, quality, or purity beyond the official requirements. Ophthalmic ointments are normally supplied in small, sterilized, collapsible tubes fitted with a tamper-evident applicator. The containers or the nozzles of the tubes are shaped so that the ointment can be applied without contaminating what remains in the tube. All containers should be adequately sealed to prevent contamination.

10.9   Labelling of Ophthalmic Preparation

Labelling:

Every pharmaceutical preparation must comply with the labelling requirements established by Good Manufacturing Practices.

The label on the immediate container should include:

1. The name of the pharmaceutical product;
2. The name(s) of the active ingredient(s); International Nonproprietary.
3. Names (INN) should be used wherever possible;
4. The concentration(s) of the active ingredient(s) and the amount or the volume of preparation in the container;
5. The batch (lot) number assigned by the manufacturer;
6. The expiry date, the utilization period, and, when required, the manufacture date.

7. Any special storage conditions or handling precautions that may be necessary;

8. If applicable, the period of use after opening the container;

9. Directions for use, warnings and precautions that may be necessary

10. The name and address of the manufacturer or the person responsible for placing the product on the market;

11. If applicable, the name(s) and concentration(s) of antimicrobial agent(s) and/or antioxidant(s) incorporated in the preparation; and

12. The statement "This preparation is sterile".

For single-dose containers the following minimum information should appear on the container (provided that the label on the packaging bears the information stated above):

1. The name(s) of the active ingredient(s); International Nonproprietary Names (INN) should be used wherever possible;

2. The concentration(s) of the active ingredient(s) and the volume of the preparation in the container;

3. The name of the manufacturer; and

4. The type of preparation.

10.10   Advancements in Ophthalmic Dosage Forms

- **Ophthalmic *in situ* gel:** *In situ* gels are conveniently applied as a solution into the conjunctival sac, where they undergo a transition into a gel with its longer residence time. The sol-gel transition occurs as a result of a chemical/ physical change induced by physiological environment. This type of gel combines the advantage of a better patient compliance and enhance ocular bioavailability.

- ***Ophthalmic inserts*:** These are defined as sterile solid or semisolid preparations, with a thin, flexible and multilayered structure, for insertion in the conjunctival sac.

- **Intravitreal Implants**

- ***Ocular iontophoresis*:** Iontophoresis is the process in which direct current drives ions into cells or tissues. If the drug molecules carry a positive charge, they are driven into the tissues at the anode and if negatively charged, at the cathode. Ocular iontophoresis offers a drug delivery system that is fast, painless, safe, and results in the delivery of a high concentration of the drug to a specific site. Iontophoresis is useful for the treatment of bacterial keratitis, Iontophoretic application of antibiotics may enhance their bactericidal activity and reduce the severity of disease.

- **Intraoccular colloidal system**: Liposomal, Niosomal.

- **Occular colloidal system:** Occular colloidal system include liposomes, nanoparticles, microemulsions, nanoemulsions. Advantages of colloidal dosage forms include sustained and controlled release of the drug at the targeted site, reduced frequency of administration, and ability to overcome blood-ocular barriers.

- **Ultrasound mediated occular drug delivery**

  Ultrasound mediated drug delivery is a noninvasive methods designed to deliver drugs to intraocular regions Ocular delivery of drugs such as atenolol and timolol, has been significantly enhanced with ultrasound technique.

- **Intraoccular particulate system:** Microspheres and Nanoparticulate.

- **Collagen shields:** In microbial keratitis collagen shields enhances drug delivery, promote epithelial and stromal healing, and reduce corneal inflammation.

- Mucoadhesive and bioadhesive system.

- **NODS:** The new ophthalmic drug delivery system (NODS) delivers precise amount of drug. The device consists of medicated drug attached to the paper cover and handled by thin membrane. The membranes dissolve in lachrymal fluid and release the drug.

11 **Suppositories**

11.1 Introduction

Suppositories are medicated solid dosage form intended for insertion into body cavities such as rectum, vagina or urethra. It is derived from a Latin word *supponere* means to place under. It is usually conical in shape and is made up of bases that either melt at body temperature or dissolve in the small amounts of fluids that are present in the rectum or the vagina. Suppositories can exert local or systemic action. The action of suppository depends on (1) the nature of the drug (2) the concentration of the drug and (3) the rate and site of absorption.

Rectalsuppositories are 32 mm long, cylindrical and have one or both the end tapered. Suppositories for adults weigh 2 grams each and children's suppositories weigh 1 gram each. Urethral suppositories are called as bougies, which are slender, pencil shaped. Male Urethral suppositories may be 3-6 mm in diameter and about 100-150 mm long and weigh about 4 g. Female suppositories are about 60-75 mm long and 5 mm diameter. Urethral suppositories for males weigh 4g each and for females they weigh 2 g each. Vaginal suppositories are called as pessaries which are usually globular, oviform, or cone shaped and weigh about 3-5 g.

Advantages

- Self administration
- Avoidance of oral and parenteral routes
- Avoids first pass metabolism
- Protect drug from harsh conditions in stomach
- Suitable for drugs causing nausea and vomiting
- In case where oral intake is restricted i.e., before surgery
- For patients suffering from severe vomiting
- Can be used as targeted delivery system
- Localized action and reduced systemic distribution
- Reducing systemic toxicity.

Disadvantages

- High cost of manufacture
- Special formulation
- Special packaging
- Lack of comparative data
- Not well researched area
- Can melt at ambient temperatures
- Non conventional form of medication (patient compliance is low).

11.2 Factors affecting Drug Absorption from Suppository

11.2.1 Physiological Factor

Rectum is a part of colon which is 15 to 20 cm long. The rectal wall is formed by an epithelium which is one cell layer thick, and is composed of cylindrical cell and consists of goblet cells which secretes mucus. When rectum is empty of fecal material, it contains only 2-3 mL of inert mucous fluid.

(a) *Circulation*: The lower hemorrhoidal vein surrounding the colon and the rectum enter into the inferior vena cava and thus bypass the liver and initiates the absorption. The upper hemorhoidal vein connects with the portal veins leading to the liver. (Figure 11.1). Lymphatic circulation also assists in the absorption of rectally administered drug.

(b) *pH of the rectal mucosa*: pH of the rectal mucosa plays an important role in rectal absorption. Rat colon has a pH of about 6.8. Rectal fluids have no buffer capacity. Absorption of acidic drug increases when pH of surrounding fluid is lowered. Weaker acids and bases are more readily absorbed than the stronger highly ionized drugs. The barrier separating the colonic lumen from the blood is preferentially permeable to the unionized forms of drugs. Absorption of acidic drugs will be increased in the rectum if we lower the pH.

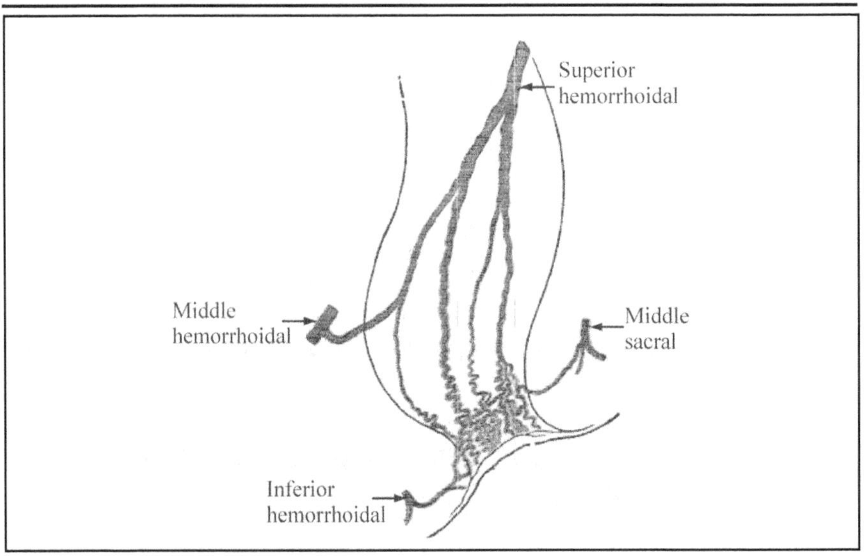

FIGURE 11.1 Rectal mucosa blood circulation.

(c) *Physiologic state of lumen***:** Amount and chemical nature of the fluids and solids present in it affects the absorption. Thickness of the mucous wall can impede the absorption. Some of the physiological states of lumen is discussed below.

   (i) *Quantity of fluids available***:** Very small volume under normal conditions (only 3 ml volume is spread in a layer of approximately 100 μm thick over the organ). Under non-physiological conditions (osmotic attraction of water by water soluble base or diarrhea), the volume is enlarged. Thus, absorption of slightly soluble drugs (i.e., phenytoin) will be dissolution rate limited.

   (ii) *Properties of rectal fluids***:** Composition, viscosity, pH and surface tension of rectal fluids have great effects on drug bioavailability.

   (iii) *Contents of the rectum***:** Faecal content present may affect the absorption. When systemic effects are desirable, greater absorption may be expected from a rectum that is void than from one that is distended with faecal matter.

   (iv) *Motility of the rectum***:** The rectal wall may exert a pressure on a suppository present in the lumen by two distinct mechanisms. First, the abdominal organs may simply press on to the rectum when the body in upright position. This may stimulate spreading and promote absorption. Second, the motility of the rectal muscle associated with the presence of food in the colon

11.2 2 Physiochemical Characteristics of the Drug

The physiochemical factors affecting absorption are:

11.2.2.1 Water-Lipid Partition Coefficient

If the drug is more soluble in the base, it will be released very slowly from the base and vice versa. A lipophilic drug that is distributed in a fatty suppository base in low concentration has less of a tendency to escape to the surrounding aqueous fluids than a hydrophilic drug in its saturation concentrations. Water soluble, oil insoluble salts are preferred in fat-base suppositories. A drug with a high partition coefficient is likely to be absorbed more readily from water soluble bases.

(a) *Particle size*: The smaller the size of the particle better the dissolution and diffusion of drug and hence, absorption also increases.

(b) *Presence of a surfactant*: Surfactants can both increase and decrease drug absorption rate. Ex. Sodium iodide for this drug the surfactant may reduce the surface tension on the rectal membrane and wash away the mucous blanket and hence enhance the absorption.

(c) *Degree of ionization*: Weaker acids and bases are more readily absorbed than the stronger highly ionized drugs. Absorption of salicylic acid is increased from 12% at a pH of about 7 to 42% at a pH of 4. For quinine, absorption decreased from 20% at pH 7 to 9% at pH 4 Phenol is a weak acid; it is completely unionized at pH 7 and at pH 4. So there is no change in its absorption when we lower the pH.

11.3 Specifications for Suppository Bases

The specifications of suppository bases are discussed as under:

11.3.1 Origin and Chemical Composition

The composition of base reveals the source of origin. Physical and chemical incompatibility of the base with other adjuvant may be predicted if the exact composition is known.

11.3.2   Melting Range

Some methods used to find the melting range are:

  (i)   Wiley melting point
  (ii) Capillary melting point
  (iii) Softening point
  (iv) Incipient melting or thaw point.

11.3.3   Solid Fat Index (SFI)

SFI is determined by dilatometry. It determines the solidification and melting range of fatty bases, molding character of base, surface feel of base and hardness of base.

11.3.4   Hydroxyl Value

The hydroxyl value measures the unesterified positions on glyceride molecules. It is a number which is equal to the mg of KOH that is required to neutralize the acetic acid which is used to acetylate 1g of fat. It reflects the monoglyceride and diglyceride content of the fatty base.

11.3.5   Solidification Point

To determine the time required for solidifying the base when it is chilled in the molds called un solidification point.

11.3.6   Saponification Value

This is the amount of potassium hydroxide in milli grams required to neutralize the free acids and saponify the esters contained in 1g of a fat. It indicates the type of glyceride and amount of glyceride present in the fat.

11.3.7   Iodine Value

The amount of iodine in grams that reacts with 100 grams of fat or other unsaturated material. As the iodine value increases the possibility of decomposition by moisture, acids and oxygen increases.

11.3.8   Water Number

This indicates the amount of water, in grams, that can be incorporated in 100 g of fat. By adding surface active agents, monoglycerides and other emulsifying agents to the fatty base, its water number can be increased.

11.3.9 Acid Value

Acid value indicates the number of milligrams of potassium hydroxide that are required to neutralize the free acid in 1g of a substance. Ideal suppository bases have low acid values or show complete absence of acids. If acids are present in the base, they may react with other excipients and they may also irritate the mucous membranes.

11.4 Ideal Suppository Bases

The ideal suppository base must have the following characteristics;

1. It should melt at rectal temperature of 36 °C.

2. It should be nontoxic.

3. It should not irritate sensitive or inflamed tissues.

4. It should be compatible with a large number of drugs.

5. It should not have metastable forms.

6. It should not be necessary to lubricate the mold to release the formed suppository i.e., the formed suppository should shrink in size after cooling.

7. It should be non-sensitizing.

8. It should have good melting and emulsifying properties.

9. It should be capable of imbibing a large percentage of water, i.e., its water number should be high.

10. On storage, it should be stable i.e., it should not change in colour, odour or in release of drug.

11. It should be suitable to be molded into suppositories

12. An ideal fatty suppository base should have the following qualities, in addition to the qualities described above;

    (a) acid value should be below 0.2.

    (b) saponification value should range from 200 to 245.

    (c) iodine value should be less than 7.4.

    (d) SFI curve should be sharp.

11.5   Suppository Bases Classification

1. Oleaginous

A Cocoa-butter: Most widely used suppository base. It satisfies many requirements for an ideal base, since it is innocuous, bland, and nonreactive and melts at body temperature. Cocoa butter has several disadvantages like:

- Fatty acids can become rancid
- Melt in warm weather
- Liquefy when certain drugs are incorporated
- Variable properties (natural product)
- On overheating, it may change into a crystal from that melts at a lower temperature

Cocoa butter is a triglyceride with predominant glyceride chains being oleopalmitostearin and oleodistearin. It is a yellowish-white, solid, brittle fat. It smells and tastes like chocolate. It's melting point lies between 30 °C and 36 °C. It's iodine value lies between 34 and 38. It's acid value is less than 4. It can easily melt and become rancid, so it must be stored in a cool, dry place and must be protected from light.

Cocoa butter exists in different crystalline forms which may be due to a high proportion of unsaturated triglycerides. Different polymorphs have different melting points and they release the drugs at different rates. If cocoa butter is overheated (above its melting point of 36 °C) and then chilled to its solidification point (below 15 °C), immediately after returning to room temperature its melting point would be 24 °C. Cocoa butter exists in four crystalline states.

(i) α form-melting at 24 °C is obtained by sudden cooling melted cocoa butter to 0 °C.

(ii) β′ form-crystallize out of the liquefied cocoa butter with stirring at 18-33 °C. Its melting point is in between 28 and 31°C.

(iii) β form-melts between 34 and 35 °C. Most stable β′ form slowly changes to ß form and is accompanied by volume contraction.

(iv) γ form–melting point is 18 °C. This is obtained by melting cocoa butter, cooling it to 20 °C, and pouring it into a container and then cooling the container in a deep freezer. If cocoa butter gets changed to one of the unstable polymorphic forms, its reconversion to the stable β form takes one to four days.

The formation of different form of Cocoa butter depend on; degree of heating and   cooling process. The following steps may be taken to avoid the formation of unstable forms.

1. Overheating must be avoided.
2. Avoid melting completely. A little unmolten mass must be there; this will prevent the formation of unstable crystal formation.
3. If the unstable form has already formed, then a small amount of crystals of stable form are added to the mass, it will quickly return to the stable state. This procedure is called "seeding".
4. The solidified melt should be tempered at temperatures between 28 °C and 32 °C for hours or days. Then it will quickly change from the unstable to the stable form.

The coca-butter possess following disadvantages:

1. Cocoa butter's water absorption capacity is low; if an emulsifier (Tween) is added, water absorption increases considerably.
2. Drugs such as volatile oils, creosote, phenol and chloral hydrate lower the melting point of cocoa butter. To counteract the lowering of the melting point wax and spermaceti are added.
3. Low contractility during solidification of cocoa butter causes suppository to adhere to the surface of the mould.

Cocoa-butter substitutes: To rectify the disadvantages of carnauba wax mixtures of synthetic or natural vegetable oils such as coconut oil and palm kernel oil or waxes may be modified by esterification, hydrogenation and fractionation into fatty bases. These processes may be so carried out as to obtain the product with the desired melting range.

B. Water soluble (Hydrophilic Bases) :

(i) ***Polyethylene-glycol mixtures***: Also known as carbowax and polyglycols. Chemically, they are long-chain polymers of ethylene oxide. They exist as liquids when their average molecular weights range from 200-600. They exist as wax-like solids when their average molecular weights are above 1000. Their water solubility, Hygroscopicity, and vapour pressure decrease with increasing average molecular weights. They may be prepared by both molding as well as cold compression methods.

Advantages

1. They do not hydrolyze.

2. They do not decompose.

3. They are physiologically inert.

4. They are not susceptible to microbial decomposition.

5. Do not require lubrication.

Examples of formulas using polyethylene glycols are summarized in Table 11.1.

TABLE 11.1

Composition of PEG based suppository bases

Sr. No	Bases	Composition of bases	
		Base 1	Base 2
1	PEG-1000	96%	75%
2	PEG-4000	4%	25%

The characteristics of both the PEG based bases are given below:

(a) Base-1

- Lower melting (Need refrigeration in summer) point
- Rapid drug release

(b) Base-2

- High melting point
- Slower drug release

The disadvantage of these bases is irritation, caused when water is drawn from mucosa which causes discomfort. Hence, polyethylene glycol suppositories are dipped in water before insertion, to avoid irritation to mucous membranes.

(ii) *Glycerinated gelatine*: Glycerinated gelatin suppositories melt/dissolve in the fluids in the body cavity in which they are inserted. These suppositories are vulnerable to microbial growth, so preservatives are added to them and they are stored in a cool place. Time taken to dissolve depend on:

- The percentage of glycerin, gelatin and that of water
- Nature of the gelatin used and on the chemical reaction of the drug with gelatin.

(a) *Glycerin Suppositories*: The composition is given in Table 11.2.

TABLE 11.2

Composition of glycerin suppositories

Sr. No.	Composition	Quantity taken (g)
1	Glycerin	91
2	Sodium Stearate	9
3	Purified water	To make 1000 g

Procedure

1. Heat the glycerin to about 120 °C.
2. Dissolve sodium stearate in the heated glycerin with gentle stirring.
3. Add the purified water and mix.
4. Pour the hot mixture into a mold.

TABLE 11.3

Composition of Glycerinated Gelatin Suppositories

Sr. No.	Composition	Quantity taken (g)
1	Glycerin	20
2	Gelatin	20
3	purified water	To make 1000 g

C. Water Dispersible: Non ionic surface active materials, related chemically to polyethylene glycols can be used for formulating both water soluble and oil soluble drugs. E.g. polyoxyethylene sorbitan fatty acid esters (Tweens), polyoxyethylene stearates (Myrj) and Sorbitan fatty acid esters (Span and Arlacel).

Advantages

1. These can be handled and stored at elevated temperatures.
2. They have broad drug compatibility.
3. They are not vulnerable to microbial growth.
4. They are nontoxic.

Disadvantages

1. Interaction of drugs with surface active agents decreases therapeutic activity.

11.6 Types of Suppositories

The suppositories are categorized in three different forms;

- Compressed tablets
- Layered suppositories
- Molded suppositories

11.7 Methodology for Manufacturing of Suppositories

Four methods that are used to manufacture the suppositories are discussed here:

1. *Molding by hand*: By rolling in to desired shape and size. Hand molding is useful when we are preparing a small number of suppositories.

   (a) *Calibration of mould*:

      (i) Determine the volume of each cell in mold

         - Pour in base & solidify
         - Weigh base from each cell
         - Put in beaker & melt to get volume
         - Calculate weight and volume of each cell

TABLE 11.4

Densities of different base

Material	ρ (g/mL)	Mass (g)
PEG 400	1.125	2.26
Cocoa Butter	0.86	1.72

Density Factors

Dose Calculation

1. Calibrate mould
2. Calculate amount of the drug
3. Calculate total suppository weight (drug + base)
4. Calculate base needed by difference

Density Factors – Cocoa Butter

1 gm of cocoa butter = x gm of drug

Use "Density Factors" to calculate amount of base displaced by drug

TABLE 11.5

Density factors of different drugs

Drug	DF
Aspirin	1.3
Barbital	1.2
Bismuth salicylate	4.5
Chloral hydrate	1.3
Cocaine HCl	1.3
Codeine phosphate	1.1
Diphenhydramine HCl	1.3
Morphine HCl	1.6
Phenobarbital	1.2
Zinc Oxide	4.0

E.g: Calculation of a given formula

Aspirin -	100 mg
Cocoa Butter	q.s.

Calculations

Mold calibration 2 g/cavity

Aspirin 8 × 100 mg = 800 mg

Total 8 × 2 g = 16 gm

0.8 g Aspirin × (1 g Cocoa butter/1.3 Aspirin) = 0.615

Amount of Base required: 16 g – 0.615 g = 15.38 g

2. *Compression*: Compression moulding is a method of preparing suppositories from a mixed mass of grated suppository base and medicaments which is forced into a special compression mold using suppository making machines. The suppository base and the other ingredients are combined by thorough mixing. The friction of the process causes the base to soften into a paste like consistency. It gives suppositories that are more elegant than hand molded suppositories. In this method sedimentation of solids in the base is prevented.

Disadvantages

1. Air entrapment may take place.
2. This air may cause weight variation.
3. The drug and/or the base may be oxidized by this air.

3. *Pour moulding*: Poorly packed suppositories may give rise to staining, breakage or deformation by melting.

4. *Compression in a tablet machine*:

Advantages

(a) High production rate.
(b) No removal by scrapping is necessary.
(c) No bulk handling.
(d) No storage of unwrapped suppositories.

Disadvantages

(a) The shape of the suppository changes with mold shape.

(b) Depression formation in the rear of the suppository since no scraping takes place.

11.8   Problems in Formulation

11.8.1   Water in Suppositories

Water present in suppositories may cause certain problems such as:

(a) Water accelerates oxidation of fats.
(b) Due to the evaporation of water, the drugs crystallize out.
(c) Chemical reaction occurs between drugs and the components of suppositories in the presence of water.
(d) Bacterial/fungal growth may be a problem.

11.8.2 Hygroscopicity

Glycerogelatin suppositories lose moisture in dry climates and absorb moisture in humid conditions so need careful storage. Hygroscopicity of glycerogelatin suppositories lead to dehydration of intestinal mucosa which cause irritation.

The Hygroscopicity of polyethylene glycol bases depends on the chain length of the molecule. As the molecular weight of these ethylene oxide polymers Increases the Hygroscopicity decreases.

11.8.3 Drug-Excipient Incompatibility

Incompatibilities exist between polyethylene glycol base and some drugs. Sodium barbital and salicylic acid crystallize out of polyethylene glycol. High concentrations of salicylic acid soften polyethylene glycol to an ointment like consistency.

Penicillin G is stable in cocoa butter and other fatty bases. It decomposes in polyethylene glycol bases. The reduction in melting point caused by addition of certain drugs such as volatile oils, phenol or chloral hydrate to cocoa butter suppositories.

11.8.4 Viscosity

When the base has low viscosity, sedimentation of the drug is a problem. 2% aluminium monostearate may be added to increase the viscosity of the base. Cetyl and stearyl alcohols or stearic acid are added to improve the consistency of suppositories.

11.8.5 Brittleness

Cocoa butter suppositories are elastic and not brittle. Synthetic fat bases are brittle. This problem can be overcome by keeping the temperature difference between the melted base and the mold as small as possible. Materials that impart plasticity to a fat and make them less brittle are small amounts of Tween 80, castor oil, glycerin or propylene glycol.

11.8.6 Density

Density of the base, the drug, the volume of the mould and whether the base is having the property of volume contraction are all important. They all determine the weight of the suppository.

11.8.7   Volume Contraction

On solidification the volume of the suppository decreases. The mass of the suppository pulls away from the sides of the mould. This contraction helps the suppository to easily slip away from the mould, preventing the need for a lubricating agent. Sometimes when the suppository mass is contracting, a hole forms at the open end. This gives an inelegant appearance to the suppository. Weight variation among suppositories is also likely to occur. This contraction can be minimized by pouring the suppository mass slightly above its congealing temperature into a mould warmed to about the same temperature. Another way to overcome this problem is to overfill the molds.

11.8.8   Rancidity

The unsaturated fatty acids in the suppository bases undergo auto oxidation and decomposition. These products have strong, unpleasant odours. The lower the content of unsaturated fatty acids in a base, the higher is its resistance to rancidity.

11.8.9   Weight and Volume Control

Factors influencing the weight, volume and the amount of active ingredient in each suppository are:

1. Concentration of the drug in the mass
2. Volume of the mould cavity
3. The specific gravity of the base
4. Volume variation between moulds
5. Weight variation between suppositories due to the inconsistencies in the manufacturing process. The upper limit for the weight variation in suppositories is ± 5%.

Displacement Factor: The displacement value may be defined as, the number of parts by weight of medicament that displaces one part by weight of the base. The volume of suppositories from a particular mould will be constant but the weight will vary because the densities of the medicaments usually differ from the density of the base, and hence the density of the medicament will affect the amount of the base required for each suppository.

The displacement factor is derived from the following equations;

$$f = 100 \, (E - G)/G.X + 1 \qquad .....(11.1)$$

E- Weight of pure base suppository

G-Weight of suppository with X% drug

Lubrication of Moulds: Some widely used lubricating agents are mineral oils, aqueous solution of SLS, alcohol and tincture of green soap. These are applied by wiping, brushing or spraying. e.g: for cocoa butter lubricant is soap solution. For glycerinated gelatin, lubricant commonly used is mineral oil.

11.9   Testing of Suppositories

For appearance tests are conducted uniformity of mix, drug content, melting range and fragility tests.

11.9.1   Appearance

All the suppositories should be uniform in size and shape. They should have elegant appearance. Color and the surface characteristics of the suppository are relatively easy to assess. It is important to check for the absence of fissuring, pitting, fat blooming, exudation, sedimentation, and the migration of the active ingredients.

11.9.2   Test of Physical Strength

Tensile strength of suppositories is measured to assess their ability to withstand the rigors of normal handling. The apparatus used is called as breaking test apparatus. It consists of a double-wall chamber. Through the walls of the chamber, water is pumped. The inner chamber consists of a disc which holds the suppositories. To this disc, a rod is attached. The other end of the rod consists of another disc on which weights are placed. On the first disc the test suppository is placed. On the second disc a 600 g weight is placed. At 1-minute interval, 200 g weights are added till the suppository crumbles. All the weights used are added which gives the tensile strength. Likewise, few more suppositories are tested and the average tensile strength is calculated. Tensile strength indicates the maximum force which the suppository can withstand during production, packing and handling. Large tensile strength indicates less tendency to fracture.

11.9.3   Melting Range Test

This determines the time taken by an entire suppository to melt when it is immersed in a constant temperature bath at 37 °C. This is also known as the macro melting range test. In the micromelting range test the melting range of the fatty base can be determined only by   capillary tubes. For determination of the macromelting range United State Pharmacopoeia (USP) tablet disintegration apparatus is used.

Both macromelting range and micromelting range are determined.

(a) **Macromelting range:** It is a measure of the thermal stability of the suppository. This determines the time taken by an entire suppository to melt when it is immersed in a constant temperature bath at 37 °C. The test is conducted using the tablet disintegration apparatus.

(b) **Micromelting range:** The melting range of the fatty base is measured in capillary tubes.

11.9.4   Liquefaction Time or Softening Time Test

Softening time is the time for which the suppository melts completely at a definite temperature. This test measures the softening time of suppositories which indicates the hardness of the base. The time taken for the glass rod to go through the suppository and reach the constriction is known as the liquefaction time or softening time. In this test a U tube is partially immersed in a constant temperature bath and is maintained at a temperature between 35 to 37 °C. There is a constriction in the tube in which the suppository is kept and above the suppository, a glass rod is kept. Another apparatus is there for finding "softening time" which mimics *in vivo* conditions. It uses a cellophane tube, and the temperature is maintained by water circulation. Time taken for the suppository to melt is noted.

11.9.5   Breaking Test

The breaking test is used to measure the fragility or brittleness of suppository. A double walled chamber consisting of a glass rod with disc is used and weights are placed on the disc. The weight at which the suppository collapses is the breaking point.

11.9.6 Dissolution Testing

In vitro release of the rug from the suppository has always posed a problem, owing to melting, deformation and dispersion in the dissolution medium. Dissolution testing methods include the paddle method, basket method, membrane diffusion method/dialysis method, and the continuous flow/bead method.

(a) ***In-vitro test***: The test conditions should be similar to those inside the human body. The dissolution apparatus is used which consists of simulated gastric and simulated intestinal fluids. Definite numbers of suppositories are placed in the apparatus. Aliquot portions of the dissolution medium are withdrawn at definite intervals of time and drug uptake is measured using a U.V spectrophotometer.

(b) ***In-vivo test***: This test is carried in animals or human volunteers. The suppository is placed in the intended body cavity. At regular intervals of time, blood samples are collected and the amount of drug present is determined.

11.9.7 Test of Uniformity of Drug Content

This test is to assess the uniformity of the mixed suppository mass. Different suppositories are assayed for the drug. All the suppositories should contain the same labelled quantity of the drug.

Unless otherwise specified in the individual monograph, the requirements for dosage uniformity are met if the amount of the drug substance in each of the 10 dosage units as determined from the content uniformity method lies within the range of 85.0% to 115.0% of the label claim. If 1 unit is outside the range of 85.0% to 115.0% of label claim, and no unit is outside the range of 75.0% to 125.0% of label claim, test 20 additional units. The requirements are met if not more than 1 unit of the 30 is outside the range of 85.0% to 115.0% of label claim, and no unit is outside the range of 75.0% to 125.0% of label claim.

11.9.8 Stability

Storage stability studies are generally conducted at 4 °C and at room temperature. Cocoa butter suppositories on storage form a white powdery deposit on the surface (Bloom). This can be avoided by storing the suppositories at uniform cool temperatures and by wrapping them in foils.

Fat based suppositories on storage show upward shift in melting range due to slow crystallization to the more stable polymorphic forms of the base (Hard). The softening time test and differential scanning calorimetry can be used as stability indicating test methods. If the suppository contains an acid, the foil wrapping may be attacked and it may develop pinholes. Stability studies should also include anticipated problems resulting from the shipment. Suppositories are often shipped by the desired transport facilities to several areas in the countries to test the effect of handling the product in the field.

11.10   Recent Advancements in Suppositories

- *Insulin delivery*: It is an alternative, more convenient route for insulin delivery to avoid existing long-term dependence on multiple subcutaneous injections and to improve the pharmacodynamic properties of insulin.

- *Bioadhesive Suppository*: These formulations facilitate the maximum drug release and adsorption of the active principle both for rectal and vaginal administration.

- Systemic delivery of therapeutic peptides and proteins sustained release suppository.

- Anorectal trans mucosal vaccine delivery system.

12 Packaging of Pharmaceutical Products

12.1 Introduction

Packaging is the science, art and technology of enclosing or protecting products for distribution, storage, sale, and use. Packaging is defined as the collection of different components which surround the pharmaceutical product from the time of production until its use. Packaging of pharmaceuticals essentially provides presentation, containment, drug safety, identity, information, convenience and compliance of a product during storage, shipment and until it is consumed. The packaging systems play an important role in pharmaceutical and cosmeceutical areas.

Labeling is defined as any written, electronic, or graphic communications on the packaging or on a separate but associated label.

12.1.1 Functions of Packaging

Packaging is a means of providing the correct environmental conditions for drug product during use storage and distribution. There are many functions of packaging as containment, protection, information, compliance and protection.

- **Containment:** The containment of the product is the most fundamental function of packaging for medicinal products. The package should not show any leakage, diffusion and permeation of the product. It should be strong enough to hold the contents when subjected to normal handling.

  It should not to be altered by the ingredients of the formulation in its final dosage form.

- **Protection:** The packaging must protect the product against all adverse external Influences that may affect its quality or potency, such as light, moisture, oxygen, biological contamination and mechanical damage. It must preserve the physical properties of all dosage forms and protect them against damage or breakage it must not alter the identity of the product. It must preserve the characteristic properties of the product, so that the latter complies with its specifications.

- **Presentation and information:** Packaging is also an essential source of information on medicinal products. Such information is provided by labels and package inserts for patients.

- **Compliance:** Packaging and labelling may help to reinforce the instructions given. The design of pharmaceutical packaging should be such that the product can easily be administered in a safe manner to the patient. If the patient feels at ease with the packaging and route of administration, the design of the packaging may become a key factor in increasing compliance. This is also an important factor in clinical trials.

- **Protection:** Packaging must not only increase compliance through its design, but also protect the integrity of the product. Packaging equipped with a tamper evident device protects against incidental and accidental poisoning. To protect children from missing the doses, several child-resistant closures have been developed

12.1.2 Importance of Packaging

The quality of the packaging of pharmaceutical products plays a very important role in the quality of pharmaceutical products. Adequate packaging helps to protect the formulation against all adverse external influences that can alter the properties of the product such as moisture, light, oxygen and temperature variations. It helps to protect against biological contamination and physical damage. It helps to carry the correct information and identification of the product. A proper packaging makes product tamper evident, child resistant and anti-counterfeiting.

12.2 Types of Packaging

Packaging may be classified on the type of product being packaged: single dose, multiple and bulk dose, pharmaceutical and medical device packaging, over the counter drug packing (Table 12.1) etc.

Packages can be categorized as:

12.2.1 Primary Package

It is the material that holds the product. It is the package which is in direct contact with the contents. *E.g.* strip and blister pack, Can, bottle, jar and tube, etc.

12.2.2 Secondary Package

It is outside the primary package which helps to store, transport, inform, display and protect the product are called secondary packages. *E.g.* carton, boxes.

12.2.3 Tertiary Package

It is used for bulk handling, warehouse storage and transport shipping *E.g.* Containers, barrels.

TABLE 12.1

Types of packaging

Single dose	Multidose	Bulk
Ampoules	Bottles	Bottles
Blister packs	Aerosol	Drums/Kegs
Prefilled syringes	packs	Sacks/Bags
Vials	Tubes	
Sachets		

12.3 Components of Packaging Material

Typical components are containers (ampoules, vials, and bottles), container liners (tube liners), closures (screw caps, stoppers), closure liners, stopper over seals, container inner seals, administration ports (on large-volume parenterals), overwraps, administration accessories, and container labels.

12.3.1 Containers

A container is an article which holds or is intended to contain and protect a drug and is or may be in direct contact with it. Containers may be referred to as primary or secondary, depending on whether they are in immediate contact with the finished product or not. Containers may be well-closed, tightly closed, hermetically closed or light-resistant Well-closed containers must protect the contents from extraneous matter or from loss of the substance under normal conditions of handling, shipment or storage. Tightly closed containers must protect the contents from extraneous matter, from loss of the substance, and from efflorescence, deliquescence or evaporation under normal conditions of handling, shipment or storage. If the container is intended to be opened on several occasions, it must be designed to be airtight after reclosure. Hermetically closed containers must protect the contents from extraneous matter and from loss of the substance, and be impervious to air or any other gas under normal conditions of handling, shipment or storage.

12.3.1.1 Glass

Glass containers are usually the first choice for a large number of pharmaceutical products for oral and local administration, due to the following advantages:

- Impervious to moisture, gases, odours and micro-organisms
- Inert and do not react with or migrate into drug products
- Suitable for heat processing when hermetically sealed
- Re-useable and recyclable
- Resealable
- Transparent to display the contents

The disadvantages of glass include:

Glass is resistant to chemical and physical change but it has the limitations such as:

1. Its alkaline surface may raise the pH of the product.
2. Ions present in the drug may precipitate insoluble crystals from the glass
3. The clarity of the glass permits the transmission of high energy wavelength of light which may accelerate decomposition.
4. Higher transport costs than other types of packaging
5. Lower resistance than other materials to fractures, scratches and thermal shock

The United States Pharmacopeia (USP) classifies glass containers as Types I, II, III, and IV (NP) according to the amount of alkali released from the glass when attacked by (or in intimate contact with) water under specified conditions.

Type I

Type I is a borosilicate glass, which releases the least amount of alkali. Water for injection, unbuffered products, and those requiring terminal sterilization are most commonly packaged in Type I glass. While surface treatment is not usually required, it will further enhance the desirable characteristics of an already superior container. In most cases Type I glass is used to package products that are alkaline or will become alkaline prior to their expiration date. However, care must be exercised when selecting containers for solutions with a pH greater than 7.

Type II

Type II glass can be used for products that remain below pH 7.0 for their shelf life. These are frequently found to be suitable for a variety of large-volume parenterals due to the less stringent requirements imposed by their lower surface-to-volume ratios. Type II glass containers can be dry heat sterilized and filled under aseptic conditions.

Type III

Type III glass has been found acceptable in packaging some dry powders that are subsequently dissolved to make a buffered solution and for liquid formulations that prove to be insensitive to alkali. These are usually not used for those products that are sterilized in their final container.

Type IV (NP-non parenteral):

Type NP glass are intended for packaging non parenteral articles such as those intended for oral or topical use. NP containers are fabricated from general purpose soda lime glass and can be used for packaging non-parenteral formulations.

12.3.1.2 Plastics

Plastics include a wide range of polymers of varying density and molecular weight each possessing different physicochemical characteristics. Plastic containers have several advantages compared with glass containers as they are unbreakable, collapsible, low cost and light weight. The problems associated with plastic are:

1. Migration of the drug through the plastic.
2. Transfer of moisture, oxygen, and other elements into the product.
3. Leaching of container ingredients into the drug.
4. Adsorption or absorption of the active drug or excipients by the plastic.

Plastics are durable, easily moulded into a variety of shapes, flexible, often unbreakable and biocompatible in many applications.

Sources of these include polymers, additives, and fabrication agents as depict in Table 12.1. For the most part polymers are biologically inert, although they may contain unreacted monomers or polymers of low molecular weight or impurities from the synthetic process, such as catalysts and residual solvents. The additives, which represent a large group of low molecular weight substances, are more easily extractable and may constitute the major reason for undesirable effects.

Factors responsible for plastic properties are:

- Chemical structure
- Molecular weight
- Crystallinity and orientation
- Cross-linking
- Addition of other agents

Primarily plastic containers are made from the following polymers:

1. ***Polyethylene* (PE):** It provides good barrier against moisture. High density polyethylene is used with density ranging from 0.91-0.96. It is stronger, thicker, less flexible and more brittle than low-density polyethylene and has lower permeability to gases and moisture. Low-density polyethylene is heat sealable, inert, odor free and shrinks when heated. It is a good moisture barrier but has relatively high gas permeability.

2. ***Polypropylene* (PP):** Polypropylene has features of polyethylene and in addition to it, does not stress crack in any condition. It has high melting point making it suitable for boilable packages and products needed to be sterilized. The major disadvantage is brittleness at low temperature.

3. ***Polyvinyl Chloride* (PVC):** It is a clear, transparent, stiff and provides good gaseous barrier. PVC is used as coating on glass bottles providing shatter resistant coating.

4. ***Polystyrene*:** Polystyreneis a rigid and crystal clear plastic. It has high water and gaseous permeability. To increase their strength and quality for permeability polystyrene is combined with rubber and acrylic compounds. Not useful for liquid products

5. ***Nylon* (polyamide):** Nylon is strong and provides resistance to wide range of acids and alkali. Not used for long term storage of products.

6. *Polycarbonate*: Due to its high rigidity and impact resistance it can be used possible replacement for glass vials and syringes. It has qualities like high dimensional stability, high impact strength, resistance to strain, low water absorption, transparency, and resistance to heat and flame

7. *Acrylic multipolymers (Nitrile Polymers)*: These are polymers of acrylonitrile or methacrylonitrile monomers and provide high gas barrier, good chemical resistance, and good strength.

8. *Polyethylene terepthalate* (**PET**): It is a condensation polymer formed by reaction of terepthalic acid or dimethyl terepthalic acid with ethylene glycol. It has excellent strength and provides barrier for gas and aroma.

TABLE 12.2

Plastic additives and their purpose

Type	Purpose	Examples
1. Lubricants	Improve processibility	Stearic acid, Paraffin waxes
2. Stabilizers	Retard degradation	Epoxy compounds
3. Plasticizers	Enhance flexibility, resiliency	Phthalates
4. Antioxidants	Prevent oxidative Degradation	phenolics (BHT) Aromatic amines Thioesters Phosphites
5. Antistatic Agents	Minimize surface static charge	Quaternary ammonium compounds
6. Slip agents	Minimize coefficient of friction	Polyolefins
7. Dyes,pigments	Color additives	F&DC colours

12.3.1.3 Metals

Metal containers are used solely for medicinal products for non-parenteral administration. Aluminium and stainless steel are the metals of choice for both primary and secondary packaging for medicinal products. They have certain advantages and provide excellent tamper-evident containers. Since metal is strong, impermeable to gases and shatterproof, it is the ideal packaging material for pressurized containers. They may cause corrosion and precipitation in the drug product. Coating the tubes with polymers or epoxy may reduce these tendencies.

Advantages

Metal is strong, malleable, ductile opaque, and also impermeable to moisture, gases, odours, light and bacteria. It is highly resistant to high and low temperatures.

Disadvantages

Metal is not inert and can be attacked by acids and alkalis. It will corrode unless coated or lacquered.

12.3.1.4 Paper and Board

Composition: Paper and board are composed of cellulose obtained by the mechanical or semi-chemical treatment of vegetable fibers derived from wood, hemp and cotton.

Properties of Paper and Board

Paper and board products are:

- Nontoxic, low cost, and from a natural renewable source.
- Good rigidity and strength, but properties change according to moisture.
- They are easily printable.
- It has no barrier properties

It is heat sensitive, poor transparency and gloss compared with plastic films.

12.3.1.5   Rubber

The rubber polymers most commonly used are natural, neoprene and butyl rubber. Most rubber formulation are relatively complex and may contain one or more ingredients:

- Rubber latex
- Vulcanizing agents
- Accelerator/activator
- Extended filer
- Reinforced filler
- Softener/plasticizer
- Antioxidant

- Pigment
- Special components waxes.

It has disadvantage of interaction, extraction and leaching of container ingredients. The pretreatment of rubber vial stoppers and closures with water and steam removes surface blooms and also reduces potential leaching.

The types of material and their uses are summarized as shown in Table 12.3.

TABLE 12.3

Types of material and its uses

Types of Materials	Uses
GLASS	Ampoules
	Bottles
	Vials
	Syringes
	Cartridges
PLASTIC	Closures
	Bottles
	Bags
	Tubes
	syringes
	Laminates with paper or foil
METAL e.g. Aluminium	Collapsible tubes
	Rigid cans
	Foils
	Needles
	Pressurized containers
	Caps
PAPER	Boxes
	Display units
	Labels
	Leaflets
RUBBER	Closures
	Plungers

12.3.2 Closures

Closures, as primary packaging components must be carefully selected as they are an essential component of the container. Closures should be as inert as possible, non interactive and should provide a complete protection. Closure for intravenous set are made from elastomeric materials (rubbers), while those that cannot be pricked are generally made from polyethylene or polypropylene. Depending on the type of container, closures may have different shapes and sizes, e.g. stoppers for infusion or injection bottles or plungers for prefilled syringes.

For parenteral preparations, the combination of glass containers and elastomeric closures, usually secured by an aluminium cap, is widely used. Typical examples are infusion bottles, injection vials and prefilled syringes. The rubber closures used within such a system must be carefully selected in accordance with the intended purpose.

Capsor overseals are used to secure the rubber closure to the container in order to maintain the integrity of the seal. Caps are usually made of aluminium and can be equipped with a plastic top to facilitate opening. Caps also provide evidence of tampering as once opened or removed they cannot be repositioned.

12.3.2.1 Function of Closure

- Provide a totally humetic seal.
- Provide an effective seal which is acceptable to the products.
- Provide an effective microbiological seal.

12.3.2.2 Characteristics of Closure

- It should be resistant and compatible with the product and the product/air space
- If closure is of re closable type, it should be readily operable and should be re-sealed effectively.
- It should be capable of high speed application where necessary for automatic production without loss of seal efficiency.
- It should be decorative and of a shape that blends in with the main containers.

12.3.2.3 Types of Closures

Closures are available in five basic designs

- Screw-on, threaded or lug
- Crimp-on (crowns)
- Press-on (snap)

- Roll-on
- Friction.

- ***Threaded Screw Cap***: The screw cap when applied overcome the sealing surface irregularities and provides physical and chemical protection to content being sealed. The screw cap is commonly made of metal or plastics. The metal is usually tinplate or aluminum, and in plastics, both thermoplastic and thermosetting materials are used. Metal caps are usually coated on the inside with an enamel or lacquer for resistance against corrosion. Almost all metal crowns and closures are made from electrolytic tinplate, a tin-coated steel on which the tin is applied by electrolytic deposition.

- ***Lug Cap:*** The lug cap is similar to the threaded screw cap and operates on the same principle. It is simply an interrupted thread on the glass finish, instead of a continuous thread. It is used to engage a lug on the cap sidewall and draw the cap down to the sealing surface of the container. Unlike the threaded closure, it requires only a quarter turn.

- ***Crown Caps***: This style of cap is commonly used as a crimped closure for beverage bottles

- ***Roll-On Closures***: The aluminium roll-on cap can be sealed securely, opened easily and resealed effectively. It finds wide application in the packaging of food, beverages, chemicals and pharmaceuticals.

- ***Pilfer proof Closures***: The pilfer proof closure is similar to the standard roll on closure except that it has a greater skirt length. This additional length extends below the threaded portion to form a bank, which is fastened to the basic cap by a series of narrow metal "bridges." When the pilfer proof closure is removed, the bridges break, and the bank remains in place on the neck of the container. The closure can be re sealed easily and the detached band indicates that the package has been opened

- ***Composition of closure***: Closures are made of rubber, plastic, metal, and cork.

- ***Plastic closures***: The two basic types of plastic generally used for closures are thermosetting and thermoplastic resins. They differ greatly in physical and chemical properties. And fundamentally different manufacturing methods are used for each type:

- ***Thermosetting resins:*** Phenolic and urea thermosetting plastic resins are widely used in threaded closures. The thermosetting plastic first softens under heat and then curves and hardens to a final state.

Urea: Urea is a hard translucent material. Urea is more expensive than the phenolic compounds, but isheat resistance

Thermoplastics resins: Polystyrene, polyethylene and polypropylene are the materials used in almost

Rubber closures: The rubber stopper is used primarily for multiple dose vials and disposable syringes

12.4 Labels

All finished drug products should be identified by labelling, as required by the national legislation, bearing at least the following information:

(a) The name of the drug product;

(b) Alist of the active ingredients (if applicable, with the International Non-proprietary Names (INNs)), showing the amount of each present, and a statement of the net contents, e.g. number of dosage units, mass or volume;

(c) The batch number assigned by the manufacturer.

(d) The expiry date in an uncoded form.

(e) Any special storage conditions or handling precautions that may be necessary.

(f) The directions for use, and any warnings and precautions that may be necessary.

(g) The name and address of the manufacturer or the company or person responsible for placing the product in the market.

12.5 Quality Assurance Aspects of Packaging

To ensure that patients and consumers receive high-quality drugs, the quality management system must take the following considerations into account if the required quality of packaging is to be obtained. Bad packaging which is the result of deficiencies in the quality assurance system for packaging can have serious consequences which includes breakage and problems relating to printing inks, or errors on labels and package inserts.

The development and validation of packaging operations are crucial in order to assure package integrity. There should be a documented process validation program demonstrating the efficacy and reproducibility of all packaging processes. The microbial barrier properties of the selected packaging materials, together with suitable forming and sealing, are critical for assuring package integrity and product safety Both the package and the product must be tested after being subjected to these stresses. These test categories include:

1. Accelerated aging-shelf-life studies.
2. Simulated transportation-shock, compression and vibration studies.
3. Package Seal Strength Testing - peel and burst testing.
4. Package Integrity Testing - dye penetration and bubble emission testing.

12.6   Special Packaging

12.6.1   Blister and Strip Packaging

Blister/strip packaging is commonly used as unit-dose packaging for pharmaceutical tablets, capsules or lozenges.

Blister Package

The primary component of a blister pack is a cavity or pocket made from a formable web, usually a thermo formed plastic and a backing of paperboard or a lidding seal of aluminium foil or plastic. Blister packs consist of two principal components:

* A formed base web creating the cavity inside which the product fits.
* Lidding foil for dispensing the product out of the pack.

There are two types of forming the cavity into a base web sheet:

* Thermo forming
* Cold forming.

Blister packs are useful for protecting products against external factors, such as sunlight, humidity and contamination.

Blister packages for pharmaceuticals consist of two basic packaging components: lidding material and forming films. The lidding material consists of a supporting material, e.g., aluminum that has a heat seal lacquer on one side to act as a sealing agent, and on the other side an assortment of other layers depending on the end requirements of the blister package (tamper-evident, child resistance, or simple unit dose delivery). The side coated with the sealing agent faces the product and the forming films. The forming film can be a monolayer sheet of PVC or a composite of other materials or coatings to increase the water vapor barrier effect.

The forming film or composite is the packaging component that receives the dosage form in deep drawn pockets. Plastic forming films such as PVC, polypropylene (PP), and polyester (PET) can be thermoformed, but other formable structures containing aluminum are cold formed.

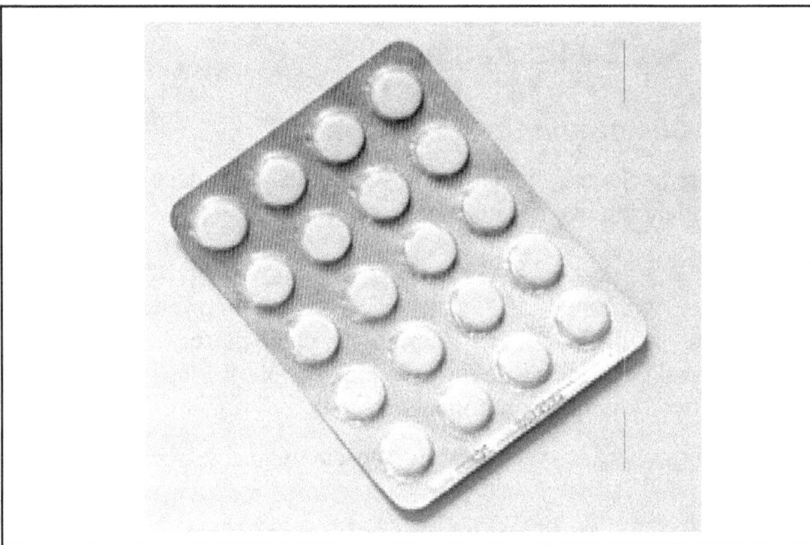

FIGURE 12.1 Blister package.

Strip Packaging: Strip packages represent an alternative form of packaging for unit-dose medication. Strips can be produced from single or multiple ply laminated materials provided the two inner plies can be sealed by heat or pressure. A blister refers to the single cavity containing the drug (Figure 12.1). A strip refers to multiple blisters separated by perforations that deliver a unit quantity (day, week etc.) of the drugs (Figure 12.2).

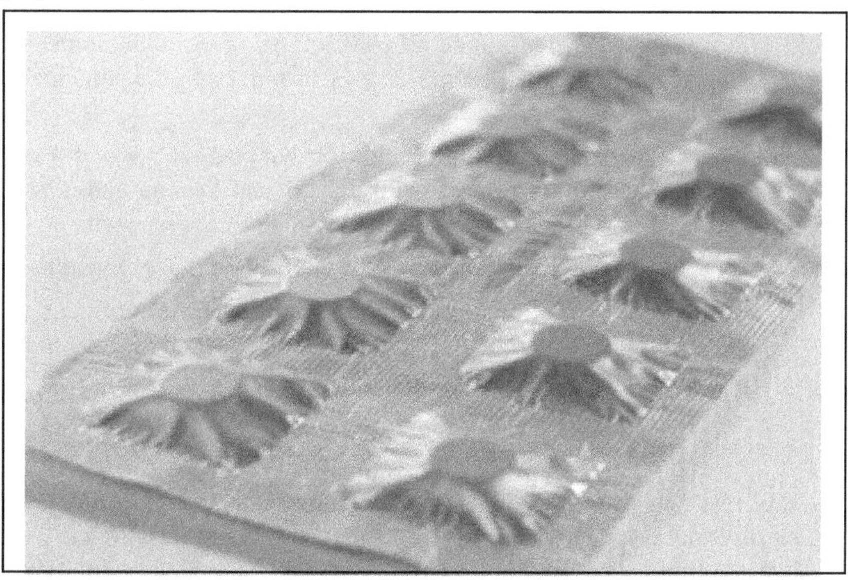

FIGURE12.2 Strip packaging.

The materials used for these packages are PVC, low-density polyethylene (LDPE), polypropylene (PP), cyclic olefin copolymer (COC), polyvinylidene chloride (PVDC), and chlorotrifluoroethylene.

12.6.2 Tamper-Resistant Packaging

A tamper resistant package is one having an indicator or barrier to entry which, if breached or missing, can reasonably be expected to provide visible evidence to consumers that tampering has occurred. Seals, markings or other techniques may be tamper indicating. To prevent the substitution of the tamper-resistant feature after tampering, the indicator or barrier to entry is required to be distinctive by design or by the use of an identifying characteristic.

A tamper-resistant package may involve an immediate i.e. container and closure system or a secondary i.e. container or carton system or any combination of systems intended to provide a visual sign of package integrity. The tamper-resistant characteristic must remain intact when handled in a reasonable way during formulation, packaging, distribution, and retail selling.

The tamper evident packaging systems are:

- *Film wrappers*: A transparent film with a distinctive design is wrapped securely around a product or product container. The tampering is visible if film is cut or torn to open the container and remove the product.

- *Shrink seals and bands*: Bands or wrappers with a distinctive design are shrunk by heat or drying to seal the cap and container union. The seal must be cut or torn to remove the product.

- *Breakable caps*: Such caps break when an attempt is made to open it. These caps provide external tamper evidence.

- *Sealed tubes*: The mouth of the tube is sealed, and the seal must be punctured to obtain the product.

12.6.3   Child-Resistant Packaging

Child resistant packaging is special packaging system used to reduce the risk of children opening the pack and ingesting dangerous items. This is often accomplished by the use of a special safety cap with locking system.

12.6.4   Compliance Packaging

Compliance packaging can be defined as a prepackaged unit that provides one treatment cycle of the medication to the patient in a ready to use package. This innovative type of packaging is usually based on blister packaging using unit of use dosing. The separate dosage units and separate days are usually indicated on the dosage cards to help remind the patient when and how much of the medication to take.

Compliance packaging has two primary purposes:

1. To serve as a patient education tool for health professionals.
2. To make it easier for patients to remember to take their medications correctly at home.

The ideal compliance package will be developed according to patient education guidelines and will contain targeted patient instructions to help improve patient compliance with the specific medication.

12.7 Analysis and Control of Packaging Materials

Advancements in instrumental analytical methods lend themselves well to the identification, control and evaluation of packaging materials. There are also precise techniques for measuring the physical and functional characteristics of packaging components. The principal instrumental techniques employed for applied packaging controls are:

- Spectrophotometry
- Chromatographic methods
- Thermal analysis techniques
- Gas transmission analysis
- Physical test methods

Quality control tests: Quality control tests are intended to check the identity of the material concerned.

All written specifications for packaging materials and containers should include the nature, extent and frequency of routine tests. Routine tests vary according to the type of material and its immediate packaging, the use of the product, and the route of administration.

Quality control tests usually include the following:

- Visual inspection (shape, defects)
- Tests to identify the material
- Dimensional tests(size)
- Physical tests
- Chemical tests
- Microbiological tests
- Toxicity tests (plastics and rubber)
- Package Integrity testing :
- *Bubble test* - blister/strip pack, liquid bottles/cap
- *Pressure decay test*-vials, ampoules, blister, pouches, infusion bag
- *Vacuum decay test* - vial, ampoules.

(a) *Physical Characteristics*: The physical characteristics include:

  - Dimensional criteria: shape, neck finish, wall thickness and design tolerances.

  - Physical parameters critical to the consistent manufacture of a packaging component : unit weight and volume

- Performance characteristics: Metering valve delivery volume, the ease of movement of syringe plungers, accuracy of dose.

(b) ***Chemical Composition***: The chemical composition of the materials of construction may affect the safety compatibility, functional characteristics or protective properties of packaging components by changing rheological or other physical properties. *E.g*: elasticity, resistance to solvents, or gas permeability. A composition change may occur as a result of a change in formulation, manufacturing process, equipment in processing conditions or in a processing aid.

12.8 Advancement in Pharmaceutical Packaging

Advancement in research of pharmaceuticals development had always been dependent on the development in packaging technology. Pharmaceutical industry, research and manufacturing technologies are continuously evolving with demands of environmental ethics and patient compliance which drive significant advancement in pharmaceutical packaging.

Now a day, many of maintenance therapies in condition like arthritis, cancer, diabetes drugs are delivered by injection, urging a need for patient friendly administration systems. These systems must ensure the potency of the drug, be tamper-evident, help deter counterfeiting, promote compliance with a dosing regimen, ensure dosing accuracy, and be as safe, easy to use and painless as possible.

Prefilled syringes: The use of prefilled syringes is an advanced way to deliver parenteral drugs, over vial and disposable syringe. Advantages of prefilled syringes are convenience, ease of handling, tamper proof, safe and a reduction of drug overfill.

Safety ampoule breaker: Safe Break is a safety ampoule breaker and it avoids dangerous glass chips contamination during breaking the ampoule. It prevents cross contamination.

Two-in-one pre filled vial: Two-in-one vial is a multi-chamber dispenser, which provides a closure solution for filling and separately packing the medication and water for injection. The mixture forms with a simple twist after removing the safety ring and flip-flopping the insulation spacer, then gently shaking the vial prior to usage. There is less chance of contamination, and it provides a cost effective solution over conventional glass vials.

Unit Dose Vial: Unit dose vial contains a plastic squeeze bulb with an integral twist off tab. Once opened, the vial's contents can be dispensed through the opening by squeezing or pouring, *e.g.* Twist-Tip™

Rx Timer Cap: The Rx Timer Cap is a pill bottle with a digital timer that shows the amount of time it's been since the pills were last taken. The timer on the cap works like a stopwatch, counting the time since the medication was last taken, and resetting itself every time the container is opened.

Ecoslide-RX: Ecoslide-RX uses a child-resistant locking mechanism that is opened with a press of a thumb with a release button in the corner of the carton. The pack is difficult for children to open, yet friendly for senior patients.

Locked 4 Kids: In this system, hooks in the pack are placed diagonally to one another, so that the tray is locked securely when it is pushed right in. Children's hands are too small to span the width of the carton and push both hooks in at once.

DISCUS ®Inhaler: It is a dry-powder inhaler that holds 60 doses and features a built-in counter, so that it is easy to count how many doses you have left in it.

Shellpak®: It is a new medication adherence packaging system; deliver pills in a calendared blister. The sturdy, protective, outer carton is child-resistant yet remains senior-friendly. Paperboard outer carton accommodates printed patient messages that remain with the medication for the duration of the regimen.

13 Cosmetics

Fundamentals, structure and function of skin and hair, classification, formulation and preparation and packaging of various skin products, cold cream, vanishing cream, moisturizing cream, face powders & dentifrices, toothpastes & tooth powders.

13.1 Introduction

The uses of cosmetics in body decoration have begun in ancient times. During that period people used natural articles obtained from plants, animals, minerals as body decorative substances. The word "Cosmetics" derived from a Greek word *"kosm ticos"* which means "having power to arrnage" and *Kosmein* means "To adorn". The cosmetics are external substances or products meant to be applied to external or local parts of the body such as, skin, face, hair, lips, mouth and nails for the purpose of protection, covering, cleansing, colouring and protection. These are mainly used for beautification or alteration of appearance. As per the Drugs and Cosmetics Act 1940 and Rules 1945, "Cosmetic means any article intended to be rubbed, poured, sprinkled or sprayed on, or introduced into, or otherwise applied to, the human body or any part thereof for cleansing, beautifying, promoting attractiveness, or altering the appearance and includes any article intended for use as a component of cosmetic".

13.2 Classification of Cosmetics

Most cosmetics are distinguished by the physical form, functions and area of the body intended for application, as shown in Figure 13.1.

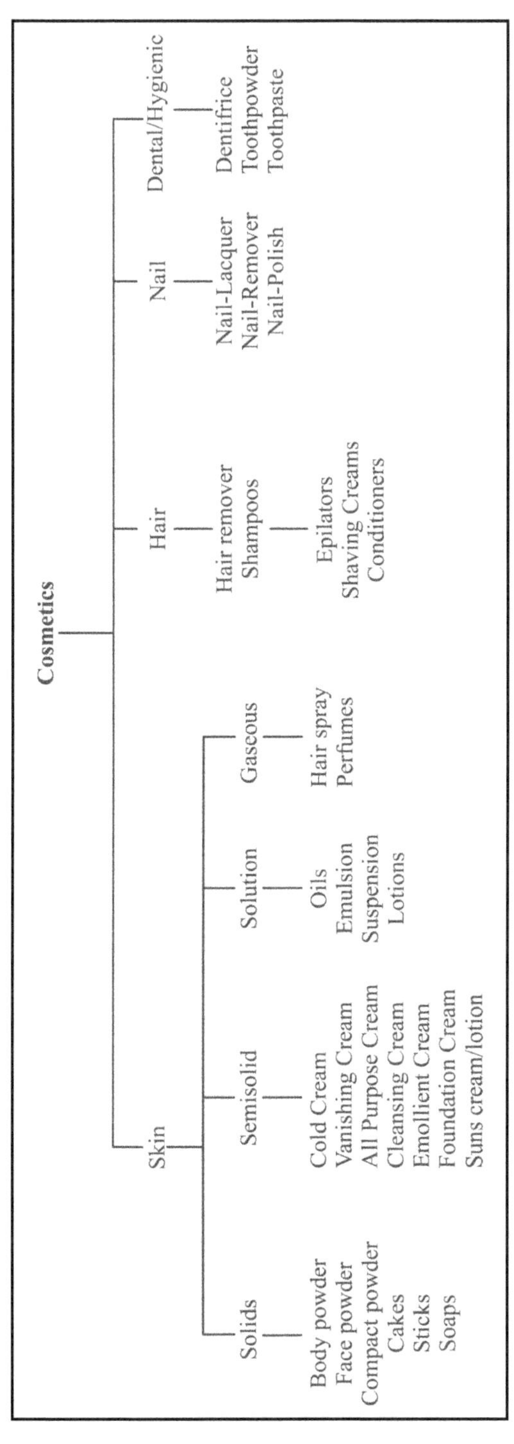

FIGURE 13.1 Classification of Cosmetics.

13.2.1 Cosmetics According to their Physical Form

A. Solids

Powders- face powder, tooth powder, talcum powder etc.

Cakes- rouge compacts, make up compacts.

Soaps- shaving soaps, Bathsoap, and shampoo soap

Sticks- lipsticks, deodorant sticks.

B. Liquids

Aquous- Solutions, after shave, Mouth washes

Oils- hair oils, Beauty oils

Emulsons- Anti acne emulsion

Suspension- caladryl suspension

C. Semisolids

Creams- cold cream; vanishing cream, all purpose cream etc.

Pastes- Tooth paste

Lotions- after shave lotions, hand lotions, astringent lotion.

D. Gaseous

Aerosols e.g, hair perfumes, after shave spray

13.2.2 Cosmetics According to their use

Cosmetics are Divided into five groups according to their use.

A. Cosmetics for Skin

Skin Cream, Lotions, Moisturizing cream, Emulsion, Face Pack, Mask, Face Powder, Astringent, Skin Tonic, Astringent, Skin Lotions, Suncreen, Sutan cream

B. Cosmetics for Hair

Shampoo, Hair tonics, Hair Gel, Hair Removals, Hair Colouring, Bleaching Preparation, Depilators

C. Cosmetics for Nails

Nail Polish and Polish Removal, Manicure Preparation.

D. Cometics for Teeth/Mouth/Oral hygiene

Dentrifrices and Mouth Washes.

E. Cometics for Eye

Mascara, Kajal, liner

13.2.3 Cosmetics According to their Function

A. Curative or therapeutic functions: antiperspirants and hair preparations.

B. Protective functions: face powders, Shampoos, Conditionors

C. Corrective functions: face powders, Mouthwashes

D. Decorative functions: lipsticks, nail polishes and eye lashes etc.

13.3 Structure of the Skin

Basic knowledge of skin, its physiology, function and biochemistry is very important for designing cosmetic formulations since; these are meant to be applied directly to the skin and its appandages.

Skin is the large multilayered organ in human body which covers 1.8 m^2, equivalent to 16% of body weight. The skin is composed of several layers such as stratum corneum, viable epidermis and dermis, and it contains appendages that include sweat glands, sebaceous glands, and hair follicles as shown in Figure 7.1. The stratum corneum is the outermost desquamating 'horny' layer of skin, comprising about 15-20 rows of flat, partially desiccated, dead, keratinized epidermal cells.

13.3.1 Epidermis

- ✓ The outermost layer of the skin, which is approximately 150 micrometers thick, is the upper most layers of skin that we can see, touch, and feel.
- ✓ The epidermis is made up of stratified squamous epithelium with an underlying basement membrane.
- ✓ It contains no blood vessels, and is nourished by diffusion from the dermis.
- ✓ Thickness is approximately 0.1 mm
- ✓ It acts as protective barrier by preventing pathogens from entering.
- ✓ Blood capillaries are found beneath the epidermis

Epidermis divided into 5 layers or strata:

- ● ***Stratum corneum (Horny layer):*** It is the outermost layer of the epidermis, consisting of corneocytes (dead cell) and is composed of 15-20 layers of flattened cells with no nuclei and cell organelles.

It acts as a barrier to protect underlying tissue from chemicals infection, dehydration, and mechanical stress. Cells of the stratum corneum contain a dense network of keratin, a protein that helps keep the skin hydrated by preventing water evaporation.

- ***Stratum lucidum:*** It is a thin, clear layer of dead skin cells located between the stratum granulosum and stratum corneum layers which is present only in thick skin such as palms and soles.

- ***Stratum granulosum (Granular layer):*** It consists of keratinocytes that become flat and lose their nuclei.These cells are responsible for further synthesis and modification of proteins involved in keratinization.

- ***Stratum spinosum (Prickle cell layer):***It is found between the stratum granulosum and stratum basale and composed of a variety of cells that differ in shape, structure, and subcellular properties depending on their location

- ***Stratum germinativum (Basal cell layer):*** It contains column shaped keratinocytes that attach to the basement membrane zone with their long axis perpendicular to the dermis.

13.3.2 Dermis

- ✓ The dermis lies below the epidermis and contains a number of structures including blood vessels, nerves, hair follicles, smooth muscle, glands and lymphatic tissue.

- ✓ It comprises of connective tissue 80% (collagen 75%, elastin 4%, reticulin 0.4%) and ground substance i.e. mucopolysaccharide 20%, capillaries, nerves, sweat glands, sebaceous glands, hair follicles.

- ✓ Its thickness is about 3-5 mm.

- ✓ The dermis varies in thickness, ranging from 0.6 mm on the eyelids to 3 mm on the back, palms and soles.

- ✓ The dermis devided into the papillary and reticular layers.

  - **Papillary layer** called as dermal papilla (finger likre projection) is the outermost and extends into the dermis to supply it with vessels. It is the junction between dermis and epidermis and mostly found in hand palm, sole of foot, lip, nipple, fore skin.

  - **Reticular layer** consists of fibers, blood vessels, nerves to sense pressure and pain. It contains collagen and elastin to provide strength and elasticity

13.3.3 Hypodermis

✓ It lies next to dermis.

✓ It composed of fatty layer of adipose and areolar connective tissues along with collagen, blood vessels and nerves.

✓ Most common cells are fibroblasts, adipose cells, and macrophages

✓ Abundant blood vessels that supply nutrients and waste disposal for the epidermis and dermis.

13.3.4 Skin Appendages

Skin appendages are derived from the skin, and are usually adjacent to it. Types of appendages include hair, Sweat gland, sebaceous glands and nails.

A. *Glands:*

Sweat glands are distributed all over the body except nipples and outer genitals. These are eccrine sweat gland and apocrine sweat gland, distributes widely in skin except for mucus membrane. It is usually found in hand palm, sole, forehead, back, neck. The secretions are very watery that contain some electrolytes. Apocrine glands are a part of pilosebaceous unit and located in the inguinal and axillary regions of the body. The sebaceous glands secrete an oily substance that protects the skin and prevent excess water loss.

Sebaceuos gland: Usually found in faces, foreheads, ears, but, it could not be found in hand palms and soles. It excretes liquid lipid to hair roots or upper epidermis. It supplies liquid lipid to outer skin for lubricating skin and reducing skin water loss.

B. *Hair:* Hair is an epidermal derivative that consists of keratinized cells tightly bound together. Hair assists in transmitting sensory information and is associated with gender identity. Hairs are found all area of body except for hand palm, sole, lip.

C. *Hair Follicle:* Lies under the skin and nourishes the hair. It is a tube-shaped sheath that surrounds the part of the hair and is located in the epidermis and the dermis

D. *Nails:* Nail is hard tissue covering the end of hand palm bone and dorsal phalanx. A major composition of nail is keratin which is tough protein. Nail grows with a rate of 1 mm/week.

13.4 Function of Skin

Skin apart from an outer covering of the body has many functions such as, to maintain the body in homeostasis, to stores fat and water. Some of the skin's major protective functions are

A. **Protection**: The skin is the first layer of protection which forms an effective barrier to the external environment invading organisms. It also helps protect against excessive water loss, chemicals, and ultraviolet radiation.

B. **Thermoregulation**: The skin acts to maintain temperature control by secreting sweat from sweat glands and thus helps to lower body temperature.

C. **Sensation**: The skin has many nerve endings that send signals to the brain to convey sensations such as touch, pain, pressure, and temperature.

D. **Excretion:** The skin helps clear the body of wastes via perspiration

E. **Endocrine function:** When the skin is exposed to ultraviolet light or sunlight, it converts a vitamin D precursor to Vitamin D which allows the body to absorb calcium and phosphorus.

13.5 Hair

Hair is a stratified squamous keratinized epithelium made of multi layered flat cells whose rope like filaments provide structure and strength to the hair shaft. Hair is made of a tough protein called keratin. A hair follicle anchors each hair into the skin. The terminal part of the hair follicle within the skin is called a hair bulb, where living cells divide and grow to build the hair shaft. Adjacent to the hair follicles are glands. The most important one of these glands is the sebaceous gland, as it produces and secretes the natural oils which lubricate the hair. Blood vessels nourish the cells in the hair bulb, and deliver hormones that modify hair growth and structure at different times of life.

The part of the hair seen above the skin is called the hair shaft. The hair shaft is made up of dead cells that have turned into keratin and binding material, together with small amounts of water.

The hair shaft is divided into three main regions (Figure 13.2):

The medulla

It is the inner center layer of the hair shaft. The pattern varies from person to person and from hair to hair.

The cortex

It is the middle layer of the hair shaft provides the strength, colour (due to color pigment) and texture.

The cuticle

It is the outer layer of the hair shaft particularly thin and colourless and provide protection to the cortex.

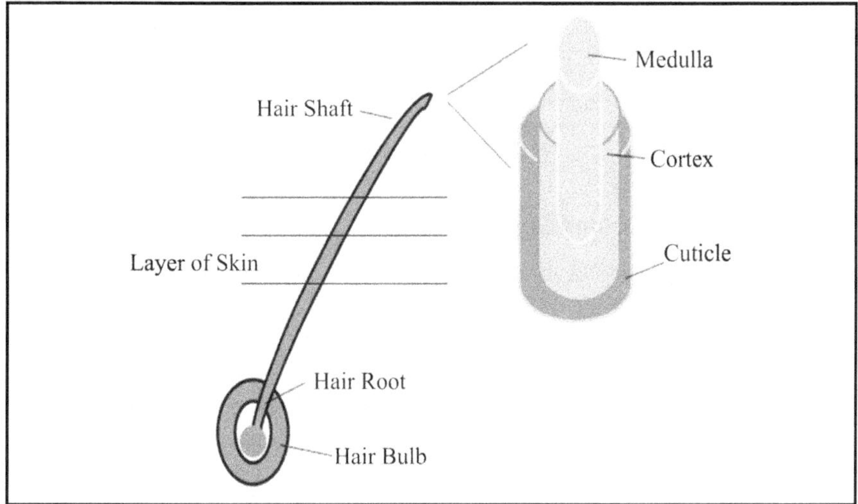

FIGURE 13.2 Parts of Hair and hair shaft.

Hair follows a specific growth cycle with three concurrent phases: anagen, catagen, and telogen, having specific characteristics that determine the length of the hair as shown in Figure 13.3:

- *Anagen (growth phase):* In this phase hair grows approximately 1 cm per month. It begins in the **papilla** and can last from two to six years.

- *Catagen (transitional phase):* In this phase which lasts about 2-3 weeks, the hair follicle shrinks due to disintegration and allows the follicle to renew itself

- ***Telogen (resting phase):*** In this phase the follicle remains dormant for 2-4 months. The hair growth stops and the old hair detaches from the hair follicle. A new hair begins the growth phase and process results in normal hair loss known as shedding.

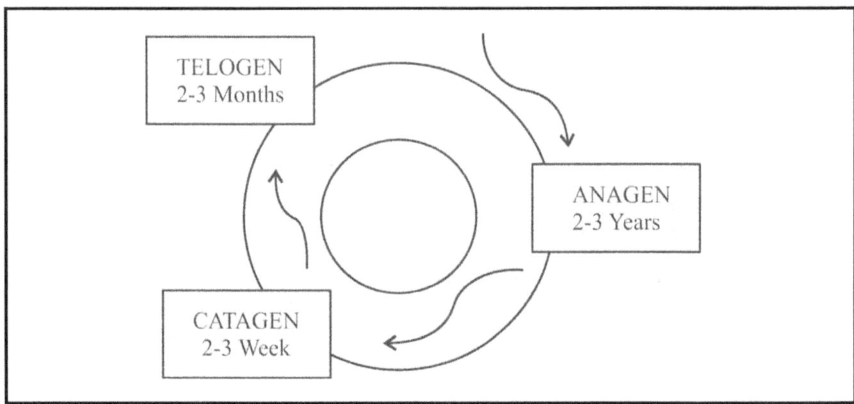

FIGURE 13.3 The Hair Cycle.

Types of Skin Cosmetics

Skin the outermost layer of the body is constantly exposed to various environmental stimuli. Also the frequent use of soaps, detergents and hot water can remove the skin surface lipids. Disruption of skin barrier led to the various types of skin problems such as, dryness of skin,roughness, scaling, cracks, itching and stinging. use opf cosmetic preparation helps to maintain the moisture and skin integrity.

Common Ingredients used in semisolid Preparation

- **Emulsifiers-** Emulsifiers are used in creams to mix water with oils.

  There are 2 types of emulsifiers, w/o emulsifiers are used for a fatty feel (eg. night & sun protection creams). O/W emulsifiers are used more in moisturizing products (eg. body lotions, day creams).

W/O emulsifiers	O/W emulsifiers
Glyceryl Stearate	Polysorbate 20/60/80
Lecithin	Cetyl alcohol
Polysorbate oleate	Stearic acid
Sorbitan Oleate	Stearic alcohol

- **Permeation Enhancer:** Penetration enhancers, helps to improve the penetration of the drug through the skin eg. DMSO, Ethanol, oleic acid, PEG, Limonene etc.

- **Antioxidant:** These are added to the formulation to prevent oxidation.eg. Ascorbic acid, Butylated hydroxy anisole (BHA), Butylated hydroxytoluene (BHT)

- **Buffer:** They are added in the preparation to maintain the pH eg. Citrate buffer, phosphate buffer.

- **Humectant:** Humectants are important cosmetic ingredients which help to retain the natural moisture of the skin. eg. Glycerin, propylene glycol, PEG.

- **Emollients:** Emollients are substances that soften and moisturize the skin and decrease itching and flaking. Emollients work by forming an oily layer on the top of the skin that traps water in the skin. e.g. Petrolatum, lanolin, mineral oil and dimethicone

- **Preservative:** These are added toprevent microbial attack of cosmetic preparation because of presence of high water content. eg. Benzoic acid, Methyl hydroxy benzoate, Propyl hydroxy benzoate.

- **Gelling Agent:** Gelling agent dissolves in a liquid phase as a colloid mixture that forms a three dimensional cohesive internal structure. eg. Cellulose, pectin, gelatin, tragacanth.

- **Perfumes:** Perfumes are added to impart a pleasant odor, mask the obnoxious odour of some excepients and to enhance the aesthetic apeal of the cosmetic preparation.eg. Lavender oil, rose oil, lemon oil.

13.6 Skin Cream

Creams are semisolid emulsions containing mixture of oil and water. This contains one or more drug substances dissolved or dispersed in a suitable base. Depend on whether the emulsion is w/o or o/w type and on the nature of the solids in the internal phase, their consistency and rheologic character varies.

Ideal Propeties:

- ✓ It should easy to apply.
- ✓ It should spread easily on the skin.

✓ It should have elegant appearance.

✓ It should be non irritative to skin.

✓ It should form an emollient film on the skin.

✓ It should not make the skin dry.

✓ It should remove easily.

✓ It should be non gritty and non staining

Preparation:

The oil soluble components (oils, waxes, emulsifiers, stearyl alcohol, cetyl alcohol, mineral oil) are heated to 75 °C. The water soluble components (methyl paraban, propyl paraban, triethanolamine, propylene glycol) are dissolved in the aqueous phase and heated to 75 °C. The aquous phase added in portion to the oil phase with continous stirring and homogenizing to assure efficient emulsification for the preparation of creams and lotions.

13.6.1 Cleansing Cream

These are used for the purpose of removing makeup, dirt on the skin and to clean the secretion of skin form the face and other parts of the body.

13.6.2 Cold Cream

These creams are w/o type of emulsions. The name cold cream derives from the cooling sensation produced by the evaporation of water, after their application on to the skin Cold cream is mainly used for skin treatment due to its moisturizing properties.

TABLE 13.1A

Bees wax- Borax Cold Cream

Ingredients	Quantity % w/w
Liquid paraffin	45
Bees wax	15
Borax	1
Preservative	0.1
Perfume	q.s
Distilled water	To make 100

TABLE 13.1B

Cold Cream

Ingredients	Quantity %w/w
Oil Phase	
White bees wax	1.5
Stearic acid	2.5
Stearyl alcohol	5.0
Cetyl alcohol	7.0
Mineral oil	3.0
Aqueous Phase	
Triethanolamine	2.0
Propylene glycol	5.0
Methyl paraban	0.01
Propyl paraban	0.04
Perfume	q.s.
DistilledWater	To make 100

13.6.3 Vanishing Cream

These are o/w type of emulsion. When applied on the surface of the skin, they spread as thin transparent film which is not visible hence, they are called vanishing creams.

TABLE 13.2

Vanishing Cream

Ingredients	Quantity % w/w
Stearic acid	18
Lanonin	2
Glycerine	3
Triethanolamine	1
Preservatives	1
Perfumes	q.s.
Distilled Water	To make 100

13.6.4 Foundation Cream

Foundation creams vary widely in viscosity and are available in the form of less viscous lotions to thicker creams. These creams are prepared by incorporating powders like titanium dioxide, kaolin, bentonite and pigments. They provide emollient base or foundation to skin and applied before applying face powder.

TABLE 13.3

Foundation Cream

Ingredients	Quantity %w/w
Ceto macrogol	25
Mineral oil	5
Titanium dioxide	10
Pigments	0.5
Glycerin	8
Perfumes and preservatives	q.s
Distilled water	To make 100

13.6.5 Night and Massage Creams

Night cream are the preparation which are applied during night time and removed in the morning. Massage cream are the preparation which are gently applied with continous rubbing on the skin through massage technique. These creams exhibit moisturizing and emollient action and thus prevent dryness of skin.

TABLE 13.4

Night and Massage Cream

Ingredients	Quantity %w/w
Beeswax	10
Spermaceti	12
Mineral oil	53
Borax	0.5
Perfume and preservatives	q.s
Distilled water	To make 100

13.6.6 Moisturizing Cream

Moisturizing Cream acts by effectively hydrating the skin and prevent moisture loss thus widely suitable for dry and rough skin on the face and body. This cream helps to bind water to the skin. Emollients are substances that soften and moisturize the skin and decrease itching and flaking.

TABLE 13.5

Moisturizing Cream

Ingredients	Quantity % w/w
Oil Phase	
Stearic acid	4
Lanonin	1
Liquid paraffin	8
Glyceryl monostearate	3
Water Phase	
Glycerine	4
Propylene glycol	4
Isopropyl myristate	2
Triethanolamine	0.2
Methyl paraben	0.02
Propyl paraben	0.08
Perfumes	q.s.
Distilled Water	To make 100

13.6.7 Lotions

A lotion is a low viscous topical preparation intended for application to unbroken skin. The most commonly used emollients are lanolin and its derivatives, sterols, phospholipids, fatty acids/esters and hydrocarbons.

TABLE 13.6

Lotion

Ingredients	Quantity % w/w
Cetyl alcohol	0.5
Lanolin	1
Stearic acid	5
Glycerin	2
Triethanolamine	1
Perfumes and preservatives	q.s
Water	To make 100

13.6.8 Sunscreen Products

Sunscreen(sunblock, sun cream or suntan preparation), is a lotion, creams, gel or other topical product that absorbs or reflects some of the ultraviolet (UV) radiation and thus helps protect against sunburn. On the basis of mode of action, sunscreens can be classified as:

- Physical sunscreens (reflect the sunlight)
- Chemical sunscreens (absorb the UV light).

Ideal Properties: The suntan product should be:

- Able to absorbing light, which has wavelength in range 280-320mµ.
- Stable in order to withstand heat and light.
- Nontoxic and safe
- Non irritating.

Ingredients

Sunscreens product contain one or more of the following active ingredients, which are either chemical or mineral in nature:

Organic chemical compounds that absorb ultraviolet light.

Inorganic particulates that reflect, scatter, and absorb UV light (titanium dioxide, zinc oxide, or a combination of both).

Organic particulates that mostly absorb UV light like organic chemical compounds, but contain multiple chromophores that reflect and scatter a fraction of light like inorganic particulates. An example is Tinosorb M.

TABLE 13.7

Sunscreen Cream

Ingredients	Quantity % w/w
Bees wax	15
Carnauba wax	10
Lanoline	5
Cetyl alcohol	4
Castor oil	63
Ozekerite wax	3
Dye/ pigments	q.s.
Perfume	q.s.

13.6.9 Gels

Gels are semisolid preparation in which a liquid phase is constrained within a three dimensional polymeric matrix with a high degree of physical cross linking Gels are prepared by a fusion process or by procedure necessitated by the gelling characteristics of the gellant.

The polymers used to prepare pharmaceutical gels include:

Natural polymers: Gelatin, Alginate, Agar, Carrageenan, Tragacanth, Pectin, Xanthan gum, Guar gum

Semisynthetic polymers: Methyl cellulose, Sodium carboxy methyl cellulose, Hydroxyl ethyl cellulose, Hydroxypropyl cellulose, Hydroxypropyl methyl cellulose.

Synthetic polymers: Carbopol, Poloxamer, Polyvinyl alcohol, Polyacrylamide.

13.6.10 Evaluation of Cosmetic Semisloid Preparation

Semisolid preparation (Creams/lotions) are characterized by visual appearance, Presence of foreign particles/grittiness, pH, spreadability, viscosity and particle size.

- **Organoleptic properties:** Colour, odour, feel, Visual apperance.

- **Presence of foreign particles/grittiness:** A small amount of cream was taken and spread on a clear glass slide and was observed against diffused light to check for presence of foreign particles.

- **pH measurement:** About 1 g of the cream was dissolved in 100 ml of distilled water and the pH of various formulations was determined by using digital pH meter.

- **Spreadability:** Spreadability determines area to which the formulation readily spreads on application to skin or hair. The spreadability was expressed in terms of time in seconds taken by two slides to slip off from the cream, placed in between the slides, under certain load. Two glass slides of standard dimensions were taken. For this purpose, cream was applied in between two glass slides and they were pressed together to obtain a film of uniform thickness by placing 1000 gm weight for 5 minutes. Thereafter a weight (10 gm) was added to the pan and the top plate was subjected to pull with the help of string attached to the hook. The time in which the upper glass slide moves over the lower plate to cover a distance of 10 cm is noted.

The spreadability (S) can be calculated using the formula

S = M. L / T where,

M = Weight tied to upper slide

L = Length of glass slide

T = Time taken to separate the slides

- **Viscosity:** Viscosity of the formulation was determined by Brookfield Viscometer. The viscosity at different rpms was measured using Brookfield viscometer to know the flow (Rheological) behavior of formulation.

- **Thermal stability:** Thermal stability (at 20 °C, 30 °C and 40 °C) of the semisolid preparation was determined by observing Globule size, phase separation at different time period.

- **Tube Extrudability:** It is used to measure the force required to extrude the preparation from tube. The formulation under study was filled in standard collapsible tube with nozzle tube of 5mm opening and applies pressure on tube by the help of finger. The extrudability was then determined by measuring amount of semisolid preparation extruded when the pressure was applied on tube.

- **Irritancy Test:** The cream was applied in an area (1sq.cm) to the specified area and time was noted. Irritancy, erythema, edema, was checked if any for regular intervals up to 24 hrs

13.6.11 Face Powder

Face powder is a cosmetic powder applied to the face or the other parts of the body to impart smoothness to the skin, covering of minor visible imperfection and for the frangrance. There are different reasons for including face powders.

- ✓ Shine control
- ✓ UV light protection
- ✓ Improve skin tone and texture
- ✓ Cover up any minor imperfections

Improve skin condition

Ideal Characteristics

- ✓ It should possess good covering characteristics.
- ✓ It should remain on the skin for a long period of time.

✓ It should possess good absorbent property.

✓ It should be able to produce transparency effect.

✓ It should br non- irritating.

✓ It should impart smooth finish to the skin

Types of Face Powder

There are three types of Face powder as shown in Table 13.8

TABLE 13.8

Types of Face Powder

Types	Characteristics	Type of Skin
Light	- Slight Covering Power	Dry skin
	- Containg higher Talc concentration	
Medium	- Moderately High Covering Power	Less oily skin
	- Lesser Talc and also contain Zinc Oxide	
Heavy	- High Covering Power	Oily skin
	- Contain higher concentration of Zinc Oxide and low talc concentration	

Raw Material

Main ingredients for the powders **are** covering material, slip materials, adhesives, absorbents, antiseptics and perfume as shown in Table 13.9.

- Talc (Base/Mineral)
- Kaolin (Adsorbent/Slip)
- Mica (covering agent)
- calcium carbonate (Adsorbent)
- Magnesium stearate (adhesives, waterproofness)
- Inorganic and organic pigments (colour)
- magnesium carbonate (absorbancy and fluffiness)
- Rice starch (absorbant and bloom)
- Zinc oxide and titanium dioxide (opacity)
- Metallic soaps (ease and smooth application)
- Perfumes

TABLE 13.9

Raw Materials used in Face Powder

Type	Characteristics	Examples
COVERING	Conceal scars, imperfection of skin/pores	Zinc oxides/ titanium oxides
SLIP:	Easy to spread Imparts smooth feeling	Talc, stearates
ABSORBANCY:	Absorb oil/perspiration	colloidal kaolin, starch, ppt. chalk, mg/ca carbonates
ADHESION:	adhere for longer time	Talc, metallic soaps,stearic acid
BLOOM AND COLOUR:	Impart a velvety, matt or peach like finish	org/inorganic pigments

TABLE 13.10

Face Powder

Ingredients	Quantity % w/w
Talc	75
Kaoline	5
Chalk Precipitated	5
Zinc oxide	10
Zinc stearates	5
Perfumes	q.s.
colours	q.s.

13.6.12 Compact Face Powder

These are loose powder or dry powder which has been compressed into a cake and is usually applied with a powder puff. The basic raw materials are the same as loose powder except that binders are used to press the cake in between 3 to 10%, depending on formulation variables.

Types of Binders

- **Dry:** zinc/mg stearate, colloidal clay, talc
- **Oily:** lanolin, vegetable oil, light and heavy mineral oil, isopropyl myristate
- **Water soluble:** tragacanth, acacia, gum karaya, Irish moss,CMC.A preservative is necessary to prevent microbial contamination
- **Emulsion:** soap/ triethanolamine/GMS
- **Water insoluble:** fatty esters , mineral oil , lanolin derivatives

Preparation of Compact Powder

- *Wet method*: All materials, binders and colours are kneaded into a pate with water, pressed into moulds and air dried.

- *Dry compression method*: materials and binders are compressed in special presses under controlled conditions

- *Damp method or wet casting method*: Base powder, colour and perfume are mixed uniformly and wetted uniformly with liquid binders till the proper plasticity of mass is obtained. This is widely acceptable and used method.

13.6.13 Rouge

Rouge is one of the forms of skin colorants/beauty aid which help in altering the appearance of the skin which in turn enhance attractiveness. They are available in various shades of colours, texture and lustre.

Ideal Characteristics
- ✓ Smooth texture
- ✓ Uniform colour distribution
- ✓ well covering power
- ✓ Easy application
- ✓ Good adhesiveness
- ✓ Easy removal without residual stain
- ✓ Compact cake which will not flake, crack or crumble.

Classification

- Powder and compact rouges
- Anhydrous cream rouges
- Emulsion rouges
- Liquid rouges
- Powder and compact rouges

13.6.14 Lipstick

Lipstick is a cosmetic product for the lips to impart attractive gloss, colour and protection when applied on lips. These contain the dispersion of the colouring matter in a base having suitable blend of pigments, oils, waxes, and emollients moulded in form of sticks.

Ideal Characteristics

- It should efficiently cover lips with colour and impart a gloss.
- It should not be gritty.
- It should have long lasting effect
- The stick should not dry.
- It should be safe and nonirritating.
- It should be easy to remove.
- It should have required plasticity.
- It should have be innocuous internally as well as externally.
- It should have pleasant odour and flavor.

Lipstick contains wax, oils, antioxidants, and emollients. Wax provides the structure to the solid lipstick e.g. beeswax, ozokerite and candelilla wax. Various oils and fats are used are olive oil, mineral oil, cocoa butter, lanolin, and petrolatum.

TABLE 13.11

Lipstik

Ingredients	Quantity % w/w
Bees wax	15
Carnauba wax	10
Lanoline	5
Cetyl alcohol	4
Castor oil	63
Ozekerite wax	3
Dye/ pigments	q.s.
Perfume	q.s.

13.7 Hair Care Cosmetics

Hair Care cosmetics helps to control the properties and texture of the hair. there are vast number of hair preparation available as, hair shampoos, hair conditioners, hair sprays, rinses and tonics

13.7.1 Hair Shampoos

Shampoo is a semisolid viscous preparation containing detergent intended to clean the hair. Its principle function is to clean the scalp to make it free from sebum, dirt and foreign substances apart from preventing the hair shaft damage.

Ideal Characteristics

- ✓ It should have optimum viscosity for ease of application.
- ✓ It should have good spreading properties.
- ✓ It should produce sufficient and stable foam after application.
- ✓ It should be able to remove waste material such as debris, soil, dead cells,
- ✓ It should provide lustre to the hair.
- ✓ It should not produce any kind of irritation or itching to the scalp,skin or eye
- ✓ It should not support any microbial growth.

Types of Shampoo

Various types of shampoos are available and they are classified based on

A. Consistency:
- Clear liquid shampoos
- Liquid cream shampoos
- Cream shampoos
- Gel shampoos
- Powder shampoos
- Aerosol shampoos (Foam type)

B. Based on Use or Function:
- Conditioning Shampoos
- Antidandruff
- Therapeutic
- Baby
- Balancing
- Medicated

Formulation:

The ingredients used in shampoo are categorized as:

1. Cleansing agents
2. Stabilizers
3. conditioning agents, intended to impart softness and gloss
4. Special care ingredients, designated to treat specific problems, such as dandruff and thin hair.

- **Water:** This is the main ingredient and acts as a vehicle, comprising about 60-80% of the solution.

- **Surfactants:** Surfactants lower the surface tension of a liquid, the interfacial tension between two liquids. Surfactants may act as detergents, wetting agents, emulsifiers, foaming agents, and dispersants.

- **Foam Boosters and Stabilizers:** Used to increase foam forming tendency. e.g.: Coco Diethanolamide used as foam booster and viscosity builder.

- **Conditioning Agents:** these are used to make hairsoften and smooth. e.g.Lanolin, Glycerol, Propylene glycol.

- **Thickening Agents/Viscosity Builders:** these are added to make shampoo thick and viscous. Gums improve viscosity because of their gel like properties. E.g.: Tragacanth gum, carboxy methyl cellulose.

- **Sequestering Agents:** Used to prevent precipitation of insoluble calcium, magnesium salts in hard water. E.g.: EDTA

- **Preservatives:** these are added to prevent the growth of microorganism, fungi and molds. Preservatives usually comprise only 0.1– 0.5% of the formulation.

- **Perfumes:** these are added to inprove aesthetics.

- **Colours:** Used to impart colour, different colours are used.

- **Opacifiers:** these are added to make shampoo opaque (not transparent) e.g.Spermaceti.

- **Anti-dandruff Agents:** Removal of dandruff from scalp of hair.e.g. Selenium, Salicylic acid.

TABLE 13.12

Clear Shampoo

Ingredients	Quantity % w/w
Sodium lauryl sulphate (surfactant)	50
Sodium chloride (foam booster)	2-4
Perfume/colour	q.s
Water	To make 100

TABLE 13.13

Liquid Clear Shampoo

Ingredients	Quantity % w/w
Triethanolamine lauryl sulphate (surfactant)	35
Glycerylmonostearate (opacifier)	2
Magnesium stearate (stabilizer)	1
Perfume/colour	q.s
Water	62

13.7.2 Conditioners

Conditioners are used to decrease friction, detangle the hair, minimize frizz and improve combability. Conditioners act by neutralizing the electrical negative charge of the hair fiber by adding positive charges and by lubricating the cuticle that reduces fiber hydrophilicity. They contain anti-static and lubricating substances that are divided into 5 main groups: Polymers, oils, waxes, hydrolyzed aminoacids and cationic molecules.

Hair Conditioners are used to make hair smooth and silky. They help by replacing materials, such as natural oils, lost during washing.

Functions of the conditioners are:

- Improve combability
- Mimetize the hair natural lipid outer layer: 18-MEA
- Restore hydrophobicity
- Seal the cuticle
- Avoid or minimize frizz, friction: Neutralize the negative charged net
- Enhance shine, smoothness and manageability.

TABLE 13.14

Hair Conditioner

Ingredients	Quantity % w/w
Sodium Lauryl Sulphate	0.5
Citric acid	2
Cetyl alcohol	15
Methyl paraben	0.01
Perfume	q.s
Distilled Water	To make 100

13.7.3 Hair Spray

Hair spray is fast drying liquid preparation sprayed on the hair to keep it in place. They contain ingredients that stick to the hair to hold it in place for a specific period of time.

13.7.4 Evaluation of Hair Products (Shampoo)

- **Foam Stability:** Cylinder shake method was used for determining foaming ability. 50ml of the 1% shampoo solution in 250 ml graduated cylinder was shaken for 10 times. The total volumes of the foam contents were recorded. Foam should retain for at least 5 minutes.

- **Viscosity:** It is determined using Brookfield Viscometer.

- **pH:** pH determined by mixing 1gram of shampoo with 9ml of water using pH meter.

- **Skin irritation Test:** Draize test used to determine the skin irritation.

- **Skin Sensitization Test:** Test carried out on Guniea pig.

13.8 Dentrifices

Dentifrices such as toothpastes, tooth powders and tooth gels are meant for the cleaning the surface of the teeth by removing the food debris and plaque adhered to surface of the teeth which is the main cause for tooth problems.

Purposes

- Cleaning
- Polishing
- Removal of stains
- Reduce incidence of tooth decay

General Requirements

- It should be capable of cleaning the teeth adequately by removing food debris, plaque and stains efficiently.
- It should leave a pleasant, cool and refreshing sensation in the mouth.
- It should be harmless, non-toxic
- It should be easy to pack and easy to use.
- The abrasive character of the dentifrice should be under the limits of the standards and should not be harsh on the enamel and the dentine.
- It should not cause damage to human health when used under normal conditions.
- It should be economical

13.8.1 Tooth Pastes

Toothpastes the most popular form of dentifrices is a semisolid product designed to clean teeth and lbreath freashner. They include the following ingredients which determine the quality and efficiency of toothpastes.

- **Polishing Agents/Abrasive Agents:** The abrasives or the polishing agents are used to Polish the teeth and remove food debris adhered to the surface of the teeth. They are used in concentration of about 20 - 50% of the total formulations andn should be abrasive enough to clean the tooth and avoid damage to tooth surface. Commonly used abrasives are precipitated calcium carbonate, dibasic calcium phosphate dihydrate, anhydrous dibasic calcium phosphate, tricalcium phosphate, and hydraed aluminahydrated silica.

  They should possess the following characteristics:
  ✓ They should not produce any gritty sensation in the mouth.
  ✓ They should possess good abrasive properties.
  ✓ They should be compatible with the other ingredients.

✓ They should be harmless to the enamel.

✓ They should provide a good shine to the enamel.

- **Foaming agents/Detergents**

  Detergents and foaming materials are used for their cleansing action. These materials lower surface tension thereby promote penetration of paste and help in removal of deposits and debris.

  Should be tasteless, nontoxic, nonirritant, producing large volume of non- gagging foam

- **Humectants;** Humectants are used in order to prevent the rapid drying of dentifrices

- **Anticarries agent:** Fluoride ions reduce the incidence of carries formation by reducing the acid solubility of tooth enamel.e.g. Sodium fluoride, stannous fluoride

TABLE 13.15 A

Ingredients used in Dentrifices

Ingredients	Properties	Examples
Polishing agents/abrasive agents	The abrasives or the polishing agents are used to polish and remove food debris adhered to the surface of the teeth	Precipitated calcium carbonate Dicalcium Phosphate (DCP) Dihydrate.
Foaming agents/surfactants	They are also known as wetting agents. They acts by reducing the surface tension at the interface of the adhered materialand enamel of the teeth.	sodium lauryl sulphate
Humectants	They are used in order to prevent the drying of formulation	Glycerin Propylene glycol
Gelling agents/binding agents	These are used in order to hold the solid and the liquid components together to form a smooth paste and maintain its property. They add up to the body and viscosity of the final formulation	Carboxy Methyl Cellulose (CMC) Sodium carboxy methyl cellulose Hydroxyethy cellulose
Sweetening agents	These are added in order to improve the taste and conceal the bitter taste of the other ingredients.	Sodium saccharin Aspartam

Table 13.15 A *contd...*

Ingredients	Properties	Examples
Flavouring agents	To imrove the aesthetic appeal as it Influence consumer acceptance.	Chloroform Cinnamon bark Spearmint oil
Preservative	These are used in the formulation to maintain the properties of the product throughout the storage period and to improve the shelf-life.	5% methyl paraben and 0.02% propyl paraben
Whitening agents	These are adderd to provide whiteness and brilliance to the paste.	Titanium dioxide (TiO2)
Anticarries agent:	Reduces the acid solubility of tooth enamel.	Sodium fluoride, stannous fluoride

TABLE 13.15 B

Ingredients used in Dentrifices

Ingredients	Quantity % w/w
Abrasives	40 -60
Detergents/foaming agents	1-%
Humectants	5-30
Binding agents	0.5-2.5
Preservatives	0.1-0.5
Sweetening agents and flavouring agents	0.5-3
Water	To make 100.0%

TABLE 13.16

Toothpaste

Ingredients	Quantity % w/w
Calcium carbonate	**56**
Sodium lauryl sulphate (surfactant)	1.0
Glycerin	22
Gum tragacanth	2
Saccharine	0.1
Perfume/colour	q.s
Water	Up to 100

Preparation of the Toothpaste with Drug

Toothpaste prepared in laboratory by trituration method. A liquid base was prepared with humectants, preservatives and water. To this base binder was added with trituration. Other powder ingredients after sifting added gradually to the aqueous mixture with continuous stirring. Surface active agent was added at the end and mixed slowly and thoroughly to prevent aeration or foam formation. Mixing was continued till all constituents were evenly distributed.

13.8.2 Tooth Powders

Tooth powders are original form of dentifrice. It do not contain humectants, water and binding agents. Tooth powders contain abrasives, detergent, flavouring, sweetening agents, foaming agents.

TABLE 13.17

Toothpowder

Ingredients	Quantity % w/w
Hard soap powdered	5
Calcium carbonated precipitated	93
Saccharin	0.4
Oil of peppermint	0.4
Methyl salicytate	0.2

13.8.3 Gel Toothpaste

A gel toothpaste is a viscous, extrudible gel dentifrice comprising a polishing agent, a gelling agent and a vehicle, along with an anionic detergent or a foaming agent. Other adjuvants usually present are colour, flavour and preservative.

13.8.4 Mouthwashes

Mouthwashes are liquid dentrifrices applied in the mouth and can be formulated either in dilute (ready to use form) or in concentrated form. types of mouthwashes :

- mouthwashes containing anti bacterials
- mouthwashes containing fluoride
- mouthwashes containing minerals (astrigents)

Types

- *Cosmetic mouthwashes:* Imparting flavour to mouth cavity, removes bad odours and give a refreshing feeling in the mouth

- *Anti Bacterial mouth washes:* Mouthwashes with a primary function of Reducing total bacterial count in oral cavity.

- ***Astringent mouth washes:*** serves the purpose of flocculating and precipitating proteinaceous materials and thus removed by flushing.

- ***Cleansing mouth washes:*** consisting of water and alcohol used for cleansing and removing food debris the mouth

- ***Therapeutic mouthwashes:*** which are formulated for the purpose of relieving infections, preventing dental caries in mouth, teeth and throat.

TABLE 13.18

Astringent Mouth Washes

Ingredients	Quantity % w/w
Sodium chloride	2.5
Zinc chloride	0.5
Menthol	0.05
Alcohol	0.6
Glycerin	8
Flavouring agent	0.2
Water	Up to 100.00

Packaging of Dentrifices

Tooth pastes are commonly packaged in Aluminium tubes are commonly used for the packaging. Corrosion of aluminium tubes is minimized by internally lacquering the tubes Paste containing stannous fluoride should not be packed in aluminium tubes. Polyolefins collapsible tubes are also used. Tooth powders are generally packed into metal cans or plastic bottle with a dispensing top closed with either metallic or plastic cap. Cans are generally made of tin plated or chemically treated steel.

13.8.5 Evaluation of Toothpaste

- Composition
- Homogenecity
- Tube inertness
- Determination of sharp and edge abrasive particles
- Determination of spreadability
- Determination of fineness
- pH determination
- Determination of lead

- Determination of arsenic
- Foaming power
- Determination of fluoride ion
- Stability
- **pH Determination**

  PH of the suspension (10 gm of toothpaste in 10 ml water) determined within 5 minutes using pH meter.

- **Foaming Power**

  About 5 gm of sample added in 10 ml of water and allow standing for 30 min to disperse the toothpaste in water. The content was then stirred and transferred to 250 ml of measuring cylinder volume adjusted with 50 ml of water. After 12 times shaking, the cylinder was allowed to stand for 5 min. The volume of the foam was noted with water (V1) and water only (V2)

  Determination of foaming power:

  Foaming power = V1 – V2

  V1 – volume in ml of foam with water

- **Determination of fineness:**

  About 10 gm of sample was accurately weighed and mixed with 50 ml of water and allowed to stand for 30 min with occasional stirring until the toothpaste was completely dispersed. This solution was passed through 150 micron Standard sieve. The sieve was washed until all the matters passed through the sieve. After washing the residue remained on sieves was collected and dried in an oven at 105 °C. After drying the dry sample was collected and weighed.

  Fineness was calculated by using the following formula,

  $$\textbf{Percentage by Mass} = \textbf{M1/M} \times \textbf{100}$$

  Where

  M1 - Mass in grams of residue retained

  M - Mass in grams of material taken

- **Stability**

  The stability study was performed by after storage of formulation in three different temperatures and humidity conditions, viz. 4°C, 25°C ± 2°C/60% ± 5% RH, 40°C ± 2°C/ 75% ± 5% RH for a period of six months as per ICH guidelines.

Index

O

Occular bioavailability 249

Ocular drug delivery
systems 196, 247, 250

Ocular inserts 197, 250, 251, 252

Oil-in-water (o/w) emulsions 188

Ointment bases 190, 191,193, 253

Ointments 21, 126, 183, 188, 197

Opacifying agents 107

Ophthalmic dosage forms 197, 260

Ophthalmic preparations 196, 198,
246, 249, 253

Optimization 67

Oral route 6, 148

Organogels 203

Ostwald ripening 171, 172

P

Paddle over disk 64

Palatability 10, 141, 142

Parenteral 6, 171, 178, 200, 205,
216, 219, 280

Parenteral products 206, 211, 212,
213, 222

Particle size 13, 63, 115, 124, 134,
157, 160, 173, 201

Percutaneous absorption 184

Permeation enhancers 195

Petrolatum 189, 191, 192, 253

Ph 191, 201, 252, 258

Phase inversion 169, 171, 176